HEALIN

THE DIAGNOSIS

Volume 5

22 HEALTH EXPERTS SIMPLIFY HOW YOU CAN SOLVE YOUR HEALTH PUZZLE

By Kylie Burton and Colleagues

Contributing to this book are:
Kylie Burton
Lisa Ann deGarcia
Dr. Marci Catallo-Madruga
Juliana Mazzeo
Dina Rabo-Alexander
Laurie Hammer
Dr. Mauel Faria
Sylvia J Harral
Beth Krause
Ally Harmon
Sybil Coburn
Dr. Barbara Layne Jennings
Amy Dilena
Christina Smith
Julie Richard
Dr. Lisa D'Eramo
Dr. Christine Cantwell
Bonnie Ridge
Anthony E. Scrima, Jr.
Nicole Tatro
Dr. John Olsen
Hali Laricey

Table of Contents

Healing Beyond the Diagnosis
Vol. 5

CHAPTER 1:

We've Been Lied to

By: Dr. Kylie Burton, DC, CFMP

We've been lied to. We've been made to believe we should chase a diagnosis. We've been made to think that a diagnosis is an answer.

It's a lie.

All a diagnosis tells us is our symptoms fall underneath an umbrella term. If our symptoms don't fit a certain criteria, then we are told nothing is wrong with us or we are left hanging in the dark with no answers or relief.

Stop searching for a diagnosis. In fact, stop trying to treat your symptoms too. Stop asking google, "What causes x, y, z?" If there was a one size fits all answer, you wouldn't get a trillion responses when you ask Google that one question.

Seeking a diagnosis has failed us. Treating symptoms has failed us.

What we really need to treat is the body as a whole. We all have incredible bodies, which, like I remind my six-year-old son almost daily when he gets an ouchie, "Our body's are incredible at healing. You just have to give it the right tools and let it do what it was designed to do."

We've lost that knowledge: our body's are designed to heal. We've been inundated with tools of management. "If you have this, go tell your doctor you need this." Now it's not just the insurance telling doctors how to treat, it's commercials and Google too. Why can't we focus more on providing our body the tools it needs to heal rather than some concoction that helps us manage our symptoms? I don't care if it's a concoction of natural products or pharmaceuticals, it's still a concoction.

Look inside your supplement cupboard. How many are you taking? How much money are you spending on them? And why? Your best friend said this worked for her so you should try it too. Google says this product relieves your symptoms so you add it to the list. Your holistic practitioner makes suggestions too and those get added on.

Can I teach you a better way? I believe there is. Let me show you what can happen when you stop searching for a diagnosis. Let me show you what can happen when you stop managing your diagnosis.

Let me begin with Stephanie's story (name has been changed). It's one that many can resonate with. She's in her early sixties and can't seem to find help from anyone or anything. After finding my podcast, "Beyond the Diagnosis with Dr. Kylie," she emailed my team and explained a little of her journey:

"This has been the most frustrating process ever. I've even tried hormone therapy and that didn't do anything. All my blood work comes back normal and my doctors are thinking I'm crazy and just need an antidepressant. There's something wrong and I know it, but nobody will listen."

How many people have heard something similar? Is this you?

Other messages I've received or heard countless times from individuals are:

1. "I feel the doctors are just brushing me off. They don't know what to do so they dismiss the way I feel."

2- "Dr. Kylie, I am one of these people. Got sick about a year ago out of the blue when I felt the best in my life. Been to many doctors, had more blood drawn than I've ever had. Always normal I guess. Then some stuff showed up and still no answers. Rheumatologist just blew it off like it was nothing even though it concerned my GP. I have a lot of unexplained symptoms. It's really frustrating. I don't look sick but I am. I've become a shell of a man I was a year ago."

If this is you or similar to your story, you are in the right place. Just as Stephanie felt when she found me:

"I am excited and hopeful that we can get me straightened out. I prayed God would give me a sign on how to find out what is going on with me and I can't tell you how many times he slapped me in the face with your name, your podcasts, your posts, so let this process begin with His Blessing."

My process begins with two things:

1. A questionnaire so I know how people feel and
2. Retrieving all the "normal" blood work they've received throughout the years.

Why? I have learned "normal" blood work has a GOLD MINE of answers if you know how to read it correctly. I read it correctly and even teach others how to read it correctly too. It saves people oodles of time and money. Not to mention I am like a kid on Christmas morning when I get a good set of labs. It makes my day.

Stephanie's labs were some good ones! Here's what I found in them:

- Blood Sugar Imbalances (which leads to hormone chaos)
- A need for hydrochloric acid in her stomach (a lack of which can lead to acid reflux)
- A struggling detox system as many kidney and liver markers were outside the functional ranges I prefer to see

- Adrenal fatigue (yes, I don't need a fancy test to determine this)
- Major signs of leaky gut, as all three markers in her labs were not in the functional range
- A need for more healthy fats
- Surprisingly, her Vitamin D wasn't terrible but it could be better. I'm a huge fan of vitamin D levels being over eight— yes, you heard me right. (Nor do I care if they're over 100.)
- Gut and liver problems as indicated by her thyroid markers
- A possible need for more iron
- B vitamins were not being used efficiently
- And the big ones: bacterial and viral infections

The hormone lab tests she received were a very minor piece of the puzzle. As noted previously, she's tried hormone therapy and worked with a functional medicine specialist in hormones. No change in how she felt.

When I saw her questionnaire, I knew why. There's more to healing than fixing your hormones. The endocrine system is just one system. Your body is made up of multiple systems that all play together. We want them to play together nicely.

On the questionnaire I use, a four means the symptom is frequent and severe. Here are all the symptoms she listed at a four:
- Chronic coughing
- Rapid or pounding heartbeat
- Chest pain
- Shortness of breath
- Diarrhea
- Constipation
- Bloated feeling
- Belching, passing gas

4

- Heartburn
- Craving certain foods
- Excessive weight
- Water retention
- Fatigue
- Mood swings
- Anxiety
- Depression
- Irritability

Notice how many symptoms are related to her GI (gastro-intestinal) tract. Not one ounce of hormone therapy is going to fix that and the GI tract needs to be fixed first.

How do I fix it? Go back to her blood work. It tells me she's fighting a bacterial and viral infection. I know these bacterial infections can wreak havoc on guts and the viral infection causes major fatigue, anxiety and depression. But that's not all. Infections can wreak havoc anywhere the body is weak. This is just one piece of her healing journey, but it's a big one.

Going back and forth between how she feels and what her numbers tell me, I created a personalized six month supplement plan for her. This plan is not intended to treat a diagnosis or a symptom. Its intent is to help her body heal. Its intent is to help each system, organ, tissue, gland, cell in the body function optimally. The body is one incredible machine with pieces that work together. Each piece needs to play its role and there's so much crossover that if you're just treating one system, you're getting things wrong.

Inside her six month plan, she knew from the very beginning every supplement she'd be taking, how much, when, and why. Because that's the way I roll. There's no guessing on my part. The blood work tells me what her body needs to heal. Your blood work can do the same, if you are reading it correctly.

If you're a practitioner reading this, you may be thinking, "What if the plan needs adjustment along the way?"

While this can happen, it rarely does. Numbers never lie and when you read blood work the way I do, I can be very confident in my treatment plans. In fact, Stephanie, like many others, are able to do this on their own with just a little support from me. I'm able to help more people this way.

Here's what she said after coming to the conclusion of her six month plan, "Gut is much better. I no longer take my medications and so feeling this good without them is awesome! I just have to watch out for BBQ and spaghetti sauce. They still give me heartburn but that's it. I'm so glad I did this and I'm hoping Dr. Kylie tells me what I need to do after this six month program to keep the gut problems far away. I like the way I feel. I don't want to go back."

Stephanie isn't the only person who has experienced healing from unknown symptoms. A diagnosis would not have served her. It probably isn't serving you well either.

Liz (name has been changed), also found me on my podcast, "Beyond the Diagnosis with Dr. Kylie." When she reached out, she had just experienced her first seizure. Being in her mid-twenties, she knew this was not something she simply wanted to manage her entire life.

I've actually worked with a handful of seizure scenarios over the last year. I love to look at their blood work (like everyone else) and play detective to discover the trigger of these seizure episodes.

Since this was her first seizure, she had only one set of labs and it had been taken shortly after the episode, so in my opinion, prime time.

One marker really stood out to me: the Neutrophil count. It was 88%!!! I like to see it around 60% so this was quite high.

The blood work was taken while at the Emergency Room and gratefully, they gave it to her so she had it while at home, which we referenced. However, the ER didn't do anything about the blood work nor did they provide a report besides, "it looks good."

Why? Because they don't know what to do about an elevated marker. If they were to show you a marker that was out of normal range (and probably way outside the functional range), you'd immediately ask, "What do we do about it?" If they don't know, why would they show you? Nor is it their fault. It's the education and training they receive. They're doing their best with the tools they have in their pocket. I've loaded my pocket with different tools. It's because of these tools that I can get different results. I want my colleagues to get different results too so I teach them my tools as well.

Anyways, back to the Neutrophil count. What does this mean? Bacterial infection. Without having any other background on her besides the one seizure episode, I asked if she had any gut complaints? That's when I learned there's a lot more to her health story than just the seizures.

Remember, I don't treat diagnoses. I don't treat symptoms. I help a body in an unhealthy state get healthy again and I believe everyone can heal. She's no different despite the symptom being a "scary one."

After reading her blood work, learning about her gut problems, and dialing in a treatment plan, the only way to find out if the neutrophil count has anything to do with the seizure episodes is to treat. So we did.

Ninety days later, here's what she had to say, "My gut was a mess! So bad I ended up in the ER a couple of times. They'd always send me home without any answers or relief. My stomach would hurt every time I ate, as it wouldn't digest anything. After trying a million supplements, I did Dr. Kylie's program. It has changed the way my gut functions. I took a complete 180 in just ninety days and now I feel AMAZING!"

The seizures are still a work in progress but every time an episode comes around, if given the chance, I correlate it to her blood work.

Without a doubt, the neutrophil count was elevated again. I know one big key to her staying healthy with very little episodes, if any, is to keep that neutrophil count down around sixty and we do that with some supplements.

I would have never known any of this if I didn't read the blood work she kept getting told was normal. Your blood work is loaded with golden nuggets too if you have the right person reading it.

Now that I've convinced you a diagnosis is not an answer nor a life sentence, let me also convince you to stop owning your diagnosis like it's something you can't live without.

Be careful how you talk about it. Saying, "I have Hashimoto's" gives up your power to heal and turns it over to your disease. Be careful how you talk about your body's health struggle. Are you giving the struggle more power or are you giving the power to your body to heal?

Let me give you an example.

I received a message from an individual on my Facebook one day. It was a voice memo and I'm always hesitant to open those. This one I knew was going to be loaded.

It was from a young mom who fought severe depression with every child she's had. This was after baby number two but pregnancy number three. We've had conversations before so I knew I needed to get my head in the right space for this one. So I did and I pressed play on the message.

Without typing it up word for word, she told me about her new health concerns and what had led her to be in this state. Her voice was shaky as she fought back tears while explaining this to me:

"My mind is playing games with me. I need it fixed and I need it fixed like yesterday. I see an [alternative practitioner] this week as a friend recommended them but I was hoping to get your advice first."

8

I'm always happy to help. However, we had a few major mind blocks we needed to heal before any physical healing would take place and people don't like to hear this. Oftentimes, we want to skip this part and just want to heal physically with some form of treatment.

I jumped on the phone with her. On rare occasions I do this. She was in a very desperate situation, possibly leading to hospitalization for her depression if we didn't do something fast.

Now, I know what you're thinking. What supplement did I recommend to her? What can I give to her that'll kick her out of this state and kick it fast?

Spoiler alert: nothing.

No supplement on this earth (or pharmaceutical) would be able to fix the state she was in.

Why? She had given all her power to her illness and her recent postpartum diagnosis. I could hear it in the story she told me over and over again. In fact, I got to a point where I couldn't listen to it anymore. The story she told was keeping her in this state of depression as she allowed it to consume her and to take all power from her.

After providing her with some other options of healing, which she declined because they weren't going to fix her overnight (if you know of something that does, they're a billionaire by now), I guided her to attend this appointment she had scheduled and to let me know what they said.

I was very familiar with the mechanism and treatment of this alternative practitioner but as always, people need to experience it for themselves.

After receiving an energetic scan, her results came up with red in nearly every column—every part of her body was not doing well. According to this scan, there were plenty of reasons why she felt the way she did.

Using the scan, the practitioner placed her on a few homeopathies and sent her on her way, advising her to come back in a month and they'd make alterations to the supplement regimen. So she followed the advice, went home, and started the regimen.

She contacted me shortly after arriving back home as I told her I wanted to know what they said and what the plan was.

Now, in the alternative health world, we all have different modalities, specialties, and ways we do business. I prefer to tell my patients the entire plan from the get-go. They know everything we will be doing up front, down to the supplement they're taking each month (when, what, how much, and why) throughout the entire healing journey. I use their regular blood work to help me create this toolkit their body needs to heal; just as you've seen in the last two examples.

As I learned of this "lack of plan," I wasn't impressed. But again, to each their own. Let me also reiterate that no supplement or pharmaceutical was going to help in this scenario. She had some deep inner work to do and at this point, unwilling to even try it.

Unfortunately, my prediction was right. She gave the story and the diagnosis so much power, telling everyone who would listen about it. Her husband ended up taking her into the hospital a few days after meeting with this practitioner. Gratefully the hospital helped her create a plan and get on some medication to help her get through these rough times.

To avoid rough times ahead, she'll be starting my new "90-day Whole Body Healing Program" soon. I'm excited for her as it's all encompassing and does exactly what it says it does: heals the whole body.

Will I be treating her postpartum depression diagnosis? No.

Will I be treating her as a whole person, helping her go from unhealthy to healthy? Yes.

To get the best results, you, like her, will need more than supplements, pharmaceuticals, a fancy dietary regimen, and whatever you can do physically. She needs to dig down deep and heal her inner self. To start, she'll learn the power of story and how changing the way she tells her story will change the power she's giving to her diagnosis.

She FOUGHT postpartum depression but now she's healing. She KNOWS her body can heal.

I believe you can heal. You need to believe it too.

So stop chasing that diagnosis.

Stop trying to treat or manage symptoms.

Stop telling yourself (and everyone else) you have this diagnosis or illness. Don't give it any power over you.

Your body can heal. Believe it. Like my six-year-old son, I'm here to tell you it can heal and it's very good at healing.

Dive inside each chapter of this book and learn what those tools can be to truly heal. Each chapter is written by a colleague of mine who has become a "Functional Blood Work Specialist" and I know you'll be in safe hands with any of them.

Dr. Kylie

* * *

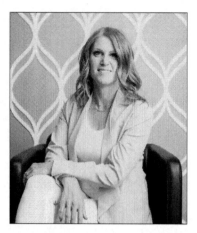

Dr. Kylie Burton, DC, CFMP, is an international bestseller with her book, *Why are My Labs Normal?* She specializes in functional medicine helping thousands of individuals with seemingly impossible health struggles, find answers, healing, and hope, even if they've been told their blood work is normal.

As the founder of the "Functional Blood Work Specialist" program for practitioners, she helps colleagues level up their patient results and build a business they love using her techniques in her programs.

Dr. Kylie hosts the top-rated podcast Beyond the Diagnosis with Dr. Kylie. Dr. Kylie has been featured on seven international radio shows. On TV, she has been a guest on Good Morning Utah and FOX26Houston, and The List (national TV).

CHAPTER 2:

Are You Cleaning Out The Refrigerator While Your House is On Fire?

By: Lisa Ann de Garcia, MA, MEd., FDN-P

How To Regain Your Laser Focused Brain The Right Way

In recent years, the phenomena of anxiety, brain fog, focus, and other cognitive issues have surged, affecting individuals across various age groups, negatively impacting their school and work performance, and overall productivity. Once predominantly a concern among the elderly, these brain-related disorders are now greatly impacting younger populations, including teenagers and young adults. This rise is not only alarming but also indicative of broader lifestyle and environmental changes. To address this growing issue, it is crucial to understand underlying causes, and adopt practical strategies to reverse symptoms.

First, A Story of Overcoming Brain Fog and Anxiety

Emma, a twenty-eight-year-old marketing professional, started experiencing brain fog and anxiety shortly after the onset of the pandemic. Juggling remote work, constant news updates, and the isolation from friends and family took a toll on her mental health. She found herself struggling to concentrate during meetings, forgetting important tasks, and feeling mentally exhausted by midday. Her anxiety levels were at an all-time high, making it difficult for her to relax or sleep well.

Terrified that her career was soon to be over, she reached out to seek help so she could get a grip on what was going on. She did not want the band-aid approach with medication, and feared its side effects. Rather, she wanted to get to the bottom of what was causing her symptoms and truly restore her health.

Within a few weeks of giving her brain and body the targeted nutrition it needed, along with some lifestyle changes. Emma began to notice improvements. Her concentration levels increased, she felt more energized, and the mental fog that had clouded her mind started to lift. Additionally, her anxiety levels decreased, allowing her to feel more relaxed and focused.

Causes and Solutions

There is no such thing as a silver bullet, but getting back your laser-focused brain is definitely possible. It is important to understand that if you are experiencing a brain-related condition, such as anxiety, brain fog, or a lack of focus, it means that your brain is inflamed. Symptoms are determined by the location of that inflammation and time of onset, like infancy vs. menopause. What is behind the inflammation? Internal and external stressors.

If you truly want to restore brain health, you MUST first deal with the inflammation and the stressors that are fueling this fire. You can do all the brain training and therapies, including speech and OT, in the world, but if you don't deal with these fundamentals, progress is either much slower or regression will occur once the therapy stops.

It's like cleaning out the refrigerator while your house is on fire.

Whether the stress is emotional, an environmental toxin, or internal metabolic chaos, chronic stress can lead to elevated cortisol levels, which negatively impacts brain function, particularly the hippocampus, a structure vital for memory and learning.

What are some of these stressors and how can we minimize their impacts?

Environmental Toxins found in food, water, cleaning products and hygiene products. It is critical to read all the labels and avoid all harmful chemicals.

Nutrient deficiencies are common because food is severely lacking in nutrients due to poor quality soil. Heavy metals and chemicals compete for the binding sites of minerals in the cells. Inflammation in the digestive tract makes it hard to properly break down and absorb the nutrients we need. In order for our brain to get what it needs, it is critical to regularly consume brain-targeted nutrition such as B vitamins, Vitamin D, and Omega-3 fatty acids, and specific strains of probiotics that feed the brain's microbiome.

Lack of Sleep. Sleep is crucial for brain health. Our brain detoxifies while sleeping, and most people do not know that melatonin is our brain's biggest detoxifier. In order to get adequate sleep, try to be in bed by ten in a dark, cool room. Aim for 7-9 hours of sleep.

Sedentary Lifestyle. Physical activity boosts blood flow to the brain and promotes the release of brain-derived neurotrophic factor (BDNF), which supports neuron health and reduces anxiety. Too much strenuous exercise can actually contribute to an excess of cortisol and inflammation. Engage in at least thirty minutes of moderate exercise daily.

Bacterial, viral, or parasitic Infections are often at the root of inflammation. Take steps to detox, rid yourself of infections, and restore your microbiome, which promotes a healthy terrain and discourages the proliferation of infections.

Learn more brain health solutions on my youtube channel: Youtube.com/wholechildlearningandwellness, where you can opt in for my free workshop "Turning Bloodwork Into Real Answers" so you can find your personal hidden stressors and healing opportunities.

Lisa Ann de Garcia, MA, MEd., FDN-P

* * *

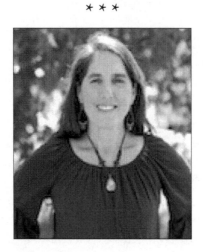

Lisa Ann de Garcia is a mom of an adult son with special needs, learning specialist, and functional health coach focusing on brain development, health, and optimization.

CHAPTER 3:

Figuring it Out the Long Way, So You Don't Have To

By: Dr. Marci Catallo-Madruga,
PT, DPT, CFMP, iNLP, CHT-P, CFN, CWC

"We do It my way, or you can get the Fu$k out of my office."

This is often how modern medicine treats the patient.

A Wake-Up Call

Have you ever felt like your body was working against you? Imagine juggling the chaos of motherhood with twins and no family around to help out, opening a business, and battling not just one, but three different cancer diagnoses. That was my life. I was constantly exhausted, in pain, and feeling like I was living in a fog. It seemed like there was no way out, but I found a way. And if I can do it, so can you. But much quicker and a heck of a lot cheaper!

My Story: Battling the Odds

My journey began with chronic pain that never seemed to go away. Despite being a healthcare professional, I struggled to find the answers within conventional medicine. Then came the cancer diagnoses. The first one shook me to my core, the second one felt like a cruel joke, and by the third, I was numb. Each diagnosis brought a new wave of fear and uncertainty, but also a stronger determination to fight.

Hormone imbalances wreaked havoc on my body, leading to weight gain and brain fog that made even simple tasks feel insurmountable. As a busy mom of twins, my days were already packed, and adding these health challenges felt like an impossible load to carry. Yet, I couldn't afford to give up. My children needed their mom, and my clients needed their health advocate.

Combine this with the chronic pain and I was unsure what I was going to do or who I was as a provider. The interesting thing: I intuitively knew that I could not tolerate chemotherapy, pain medication or muscle relaxers. So I had to find a way to solve the issues on my own.

Why? Why not try the conventional route?

I did. I was told by a rheumatologist, "Let's just try this medication. If it works, great, we can tell you what is wrong with you. If not, in ninety days we will try a new one." When I asked about testing I was laughed at. When I said that I had done the research and knew that there were genetic markers that we could look at. With my husband in the room, He looked at me and point blank said, "We can do this my way, or you can get the F$%K out of my office."

A few weeks later I had the opportunity to work with a Hematology Expert who actually did the testing. Turns out, I don't have the genetic markers for autoimmune, but I did have some others that lead to this path. The problem: She didn't know what to do with the information because it was not well understood at the time. But she told me, "Keep going. YOU are on the right track."

And so I did. It took me six years and over $100,000.

I don't want it to take this much for you.

Through sheer determination, I began exploring alternative approaches. I delved into detoxification, metabolic restoration, and genetics. Slowly but surely, I started to reclaim my health. The chronic pain lessened, the fog lifted, weight came off, and my energy levels began to rise. It wasn't an overnight miracle, but a journey of small, consistent steps that led to big changes.

7 Steps to Start Detoxing Your Body

If you're feeling overwhelmed by your health challenges, know that you can start small. Here are seven simple steps to begin detoxing your body and reclaiming your vitality:

1. Hydrate with Purpose: Drink plenty of water, aiming for at least eight glasses a day. Add a slice of lemon, ginger and Cayenne for an extra detox boost.

2. Eat Clean: Focus on whole foods. Avoid processed foods, sugars, and artificial additives.

3. Move Daily & Sweat: Incorporate at least thirty minutes of physical activity into your routine. It can be as simple as a brisk walk. But sweat. Sauna can also be helpful

4. Prioritize Sleep: Aim for 7-9 hours of quality sleep each night.

5. No Synthetics: Get rid of artificial and synthetic fragrances

6. Support Your Gut: Include probiotics and fiber-rich foods to support a healthy digestive system.

7. Manage Stress: Practice mindfulness, meditation, or yoga to reduce stress levels.

Embarking on a health journey can be daunting, but you don't have to do it alone. I've walked this path and come out stronger, and I'm here to help you do the same. One of the most important aspects of any health journey is a provider who communicates openly and often. They have to do a good intake and follow up. You are your best expert. What you need is a roadmap and a guide.

If you're ready to take the first step towards a healthier, more vibrant you, reach out to me at drmarci@agilityphysio.com or visit my website at (http://www.5280restorativemed.com).

Remember, healing is a journey, and every small step brings you closer to your goal.

* * *

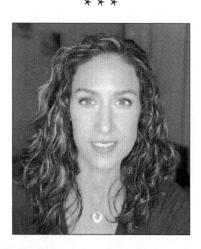

Dr. Marci Catallo-Madruga is a licensed physical therapist and functional medicine provider. She and her husband live with their children in Colorado. They enjoy hiking, swimming, skiing and golf, and one of the twins plays lacrosse. Dr. Marci CM truly believes that everyone has what they need to heal and are more than their diagnosis. They just need to remember the amazing capabilities their body poses.

CHAPTER 4:

The Cure For Bad Breath

By: Juliana Mazzeo, M.S, CDN, FMHC

Attention: Is your reflux causing offensive breath? You have asked your doctor but they deny any correlation between reflux and bad breath. You know something is wrong but you are not getting any answers. This issue is affecting your quality of life.

Do you want to stop the dragon breath? Stop the heartburn naturally? Enjoy meals with friends and family without having to think about which food is going to put a flame in your stomach?

Meet Tom, husband and father of two. Tom has been on antacids medications to stop the acid reflux for over fifteen years. His medicines were changed many times over these years, yet the heartburn and pain continued. Tom was also constantly chewing over the counter drugs to stop the acid in his stomach from coming up in his throat. Nothing was helping him.

Meal times were problematic for Tom because no matter what he ate or avoided, something would make the acid reflux worse, and the belching after meals was so embarrassing. He avoided having lunches with his clients. Dinner with the family had turned into a very unpleasant event.

Aside from the horrible acid reflux that he was struggling with, Tom also was suffering with severe bad breath which was caused by the prescription drugs he was taking to stop the acid in the stomach. Tom did some research and learned that when these medications are used to stop the acid in the stomach, the food is not digested and the body does not absorb any nutrients because without the acid naturally produced by the stomach, the food sits in the stomach fermenting and thus causing bad breath.

The offensive breath was affecting his work. Tom was an insurance agent and when speaking with clients he would notice them move away from him to avoid his breath.

If that wasn't bad enough his wife was becoming distant and could not bear to kiss him. His two children didn't want to kiss or hug daddy. Tom was so hurt and longed for the affection and closeness of his wife and kids, but he understood why they didn't want to get close to him.

Tom had tried everything for the bad breath. Different toothpastes, mouth washes, mints, teas. Nothing helped!

That year, Tom spent Christmas with his sister Mary and her family. Mary was one of my clients many years ago. Tom opened up to Mary about his awful reflux, the pain, belching, and the embarrassing and emotionally painful bad breath he was struggling with.

He told Mary he had been to all the stomach specialists, had all the tests done, had been taking these awful drugs that don't work and chewing the over the counter drugs to stop the acid and still no relief to be had. The doctors just kept refilling his prescriptions which he was told he would need the rest of his life.

Mary recommended me.

Tom trusted his sister and her recommendations. What did he have to lose? After fifteen years of taking these horrible drugs that could possibly destroy his bones, and they don't even work, and they make his breath offensive, so offensive that people including his family members don't come too close to him. He had given the medical route 15+ years of his life trying to get answers and relief and resolve the acid reflux for once and for all. All to no avail.

Tom reached out to me after the Christmas Holidays, saying he was desperate for help. **My 90 Day Gut Restoration Program** addressed the real cause of the reflux problem without restrictive dieting or eliminating every food on the planet that may cause heartburn one day and not the next.

And even if he tried all those food elimination diets, used drugs and over the counter drugs to stop the acid, and nothing worked. And actually got worse.

Fast forward a month into the program, Tom emailed me to let me know he was feeling so much better and stopped taking the over the counter drugs. Within two months of being on the program he was tolerating different foods that he had been avoiding and his belching had decreased by 70%. He also saw his stomach doctor and was being weaned off the prescription drugs he had been taking for fifteen years. By the end of month three, Tom was completely off the prescription meds and noticed that within a couple of weeks the awful offensive breath disappeared just like that.

Tom was thrilled. Not only did he feel well because now he was actually absorbing the nutrients from his food, he was able to enjoy meals with his family and he was able to kiss his wife and children and enjoy their affection which he had been missing for years.

Because of his ability to speak with people without worrying about his breath, he was able to get new clients for his business and that skyrocketed his confidence.

How many of you can relate to Tom? Have you had enough of chasing symptoms and medicating yourself for years with no relief in sight?

Simple tips to get you started:

- Apple cider vinegar (ACV)—A mild acid to help digest food so it does not ferment in the stomach. Fermentation should never happen in the stomach. Mix 1 tbsp. ACV with 4-6oz of water before every meal.
- Chamomile Tea—a cooling and soothing herb. Drink in the evening after dinner.
- Drink 1-2 oz. of Aloe Vera Juice 2-3 times per day—start slowly.
- Avoid eating late, and laying down too soon after a meal.

* Do NOT stop your medications cold turkey. This will cause a rebound effect.

* * *

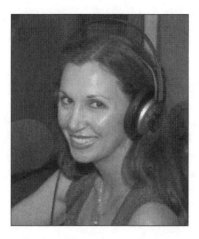

Juliana Mazzeo is a trailblazer in functional nutrition, dedicated to helping women over forty unlock the secrets hidden within their blood work.

With an advanced Master of Science in Clinical Nutrition from LIU C.W. Post and a Bachelor of Arts in Psychology from Adelphi University, Juliana combines her nutritional expertise with a deep understanding of the psychological aspects of health.

As the founder of the Nutrition Wellness Center in Valley Stream, New York, Juliana has spent over two decades unraveling complex health puzzles specifically for women navigating the challenges of midlife. Her innovative approach integrates functional blood work analysis with personalized nutrition plans, empowering women to rewrite their health stories and reclaim their vitality.

Juliana's extensive experience includes serving as the Director of Nutrition for The Cardiovascular Wellness Centers of Westbury and NY from 2000 to 2010, where she specialized in managing conditions such as coronary heart disease, diabetes, and obesity.

A respected voice in her field, Juliana is co-author of the International Best Seller *Healing Beyond The Diagnosis Volume 4: 18 Health Experts Simplify How You Can Solve Your Health Puzzle*. Her co- research on cardiovascular risk factors in diabetics was published in the American College of Nutrition, and she contributed to *101 Great Ways To Improve Your Health*, highlighting the dangers of acid blockers.

Juliana has garnered media attention through regular appearances on WOR 710 AM's "The Heart Show" WGBB 1240AM, and Cablevision's "Tooth or Consequences."

She specializes in addressing unique health challenges faced by women over forty, including hormonal imbalances, weight management, gastrointestinal issues, and prevention of age-related diseases. With a career spanning over twenty-five years, Juliana Mazzeo remains at the forefront of functional nutrition, offering hope and transformative health solutions to women seeking to thrive in their forties, fifties, sixties and beyond.

CHAPTER 5:

Your Biggest Fear

By: Dina Rabo-Alexander

What has been your biggest fear up until this moment of why you haven't gotten help for your ongoing mood swings, your fatigue and irritability that leaves you feeling less than optimal for not only yourself but for others around you? Have you wanted to find a solution to truly feeling better, to having more energy, getting more from your day, but have been told "this is just you" or, "you're getting older and this is just what happens, your hormonal, this is being a mom?"

Well, I wasn't ready to swallow that pill. That common denominator that many people, especially women, get fed when they seek out medical help for their condition(s). Maybe there are a lot of women out there who feel fatigued and depleted, they are raising their families or they are showing up in their career or doing both and they struggle everyday with trying to beat their mood swings, dealing with the "highs and lows of their day," trying to keep enough caffeine in them to get to "the next thing." Tired of feeling tired, unmotivated, dealing with brain fog, anxiety and even sleepless nights, despite being told "everything looks good, this is just part of being a mom, part of getting older just deal with it." Well I knew there was a better answer and a way to not only help myself but to help women like me.

I have been helping individuals for twenty years as a chiropractor and it wasn't until I had to put the oxygen mask on myself (remember the flight attendant telling you on the plane) that I really started to heal and understand my own "pain beneath my pain" or as I now note it as discovering the "hidden weaknesses" that make us less than the optimal human beings we were designed to be. The world today is more stressed on multiple levels than ever. As the average individual is exposed to over 700 different contaminants daily, including various chemical and environmental pollutants found in our food, the air we live and work in, the chemicals in our clothing and not to mention our homes that can be linked to various health conditions. (EWG Environmental Working Group 2024. It's no wonder our bodies, our nervous system gets stuck and can't clear the system on its own.)

Stress levels in the US from a 2023 survey from the American Psychological Association reported that 84% of adults experienced "prolonged stress with significant stress levels increased in relation to their finances, political, family and health issues."

It's no secret that most individuals who seek out a chiropractor have been to multiple doctors to seek a solution to their health problem(s). What motivated me to do what I do was because I was like a health coach. I was trained in solutions to help deal with pain and restore normal motion and function to the nervous system naturally. However, as time went on and I got busier it was also apparent that individuals weren't responding favorably to treatment. Patients were dealing with more joint inflammation, experiencing more chronic issues, fatigue and mood swings. They were not fully recovering with treatments as they once had early on. Since women are almost twice as likely to seek medical care over men (based on a 2020 CDC report) and 77% of women utilize services like routine blood pressure checks, pap tests, and mammograms more frequently than men along with preventive treatments, most of my patients were women. I was more frustrated than ever at not truly seeing results with my female patients. Somewhat discouraged, I continued to delve deeper, there had to be more answers to finding resolution to such health conditions. What were some of the true causes or weaknesses behind their fatigue, their ailments like diffuse joint pain, their feelings of anxiety and stress. That's when I discovered looking at blood work on a different level.

I found a colleague who was teaching lab work evaluation like nothing I had learned in my college and doctorate courses. It made sense, there are patterns that are apparent in common blood work that tell a story. I was my first experimental subject, I myself at the age of forty-seven had been in a solo practice, feeling myself overwhelmed, fatigued, stressed with life in general, not able to find a diet that was suitable to avoiding my bloated belly and having gained weight during chiropractic school (about twenty pounds). I was at a loss. I evaluated my own blood work results and was taught how cortisol and blood sugar were sabotaging my well-being in other metabolic areas. I resolved to commit to healing my own self and restoring my own short falls to go from unhealthy to healthy. It took some time, but through continued lifestyle changes, the right nutrients to fill in the gaps that were needed, after more than like six months, I felt I was the person I was designed to be!

I have now taken my experience and expertise in helping other women similar to myself and more to getting their life back, despite being told, "All is normal and this is just you getting older." Poppycock, I now have testimonies from others who have walked my walk and have shared their experience of going from "unhealthy to healthy," and living their best life for themselves and their family, their loved ones, and more. I teach others five key things to find in the blood work they have that can give them answers to why they lack energy and haven't been able to get answers to their GI issues and more. If this sounds like something you would be interested in for more information go to Bloodworkspecialistenergyreboot.com. Also find me on Facebook at RaboHealth and Instagram @DrDinaRabo.

✳ ✳ ✳

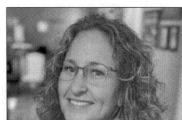

Dr. Dina Rabo-Alexander is a Chiropractor specializing in whole body healing to help others make lasting lifestyle changes to live their best life. She helps others understand their blood work to improve their health, reduce stress, experience more energy while achieving lasting health goals. She runs two successful offices and when not seeing patients, she enjoys the outdoors with her husband, Steve, and traveling.

CHAPTER 6:

Healing Beyond A Bulimia Diagnosis

By: Laurie Hammer, FNTP, NNTS

At twelve-years-old, I found myself constantly standing in front of a mirror, convinced I was fat and hating my body. It was the beginning of a nearly twelve-year struggle with an eating disorder that almost claimed my life.

My battle with bulimia, anxiety, and depression began in 8th grade, fueled by insecurities about my appearance and a stressful family dynamic. My mom's constant dieting and poor relationship with food only worsened my fears of being fat, ugly and unwanted. One night I was watching the Karen Carpenter movie and sadly thought her way of losing weight might bring me the control over my body I desperately craved. I didn't want to get fat and certainly wasn't at the time, but I didn't see myself that way. Unfortunately, this "short term experiment" with bulimia instead spiraled into nearly a twelve-year dark journey for me.

College exacerbated my problems. As the bulimia worsened, so did the anxiety and depression. I was sneaking and stealing food, binging and purging multiple times a day, and missing classes.

Eventually, I had to drop out of nursing school in my third year because I was so depressed and just couldn't study or attend my clinical's. Despite consistent counseling and joining an eating disorder support group, my destructive behaviors continued. I ended up in the ER multiple times due to severe electrolyte imbalances, leading to seizures. My life became a series of failed jobs, schools, and strained family relationships. I genuinely believed I might die from a heart attack or something else. I was in a dark, desperate situation at that time and I didn't know how to stop the binging and purging. I would wake up every day and think, "This is a new day and I won't binge or purge today."...but most days didn't work out that way and I would be right back in the cycle by lunch time. I was deeply depressed and the anxiety would just grip me as well, so much so that I didn't even want to be with anyone. I would hide in my apartment and white knuckle my way through each day and feel like a failure as I gave in to the silent monster within.

Running and walking for hours became my escape, even at 2 a.m. when it was really not safe to go for a run. I would have drank gasoline at that time if someone would have told me it would stop the binging and purging and make the depression and anxiety go away. I tried a lot of things to stop the cycle: counseling, smoking pot, drinking a couple beers at night, going to bed at 6 p.m.... but nothing would stop the cycle. I would still find myself at the donut shop drive up window at 11 p.m. and the vicious cycle would continue.

A turning point came when a nursing professor and friend sent me an article suggesting that I might be "addicted to what I was allergic to" and that allergy could be depleting my brain. This powerful article led me to an outpatient clinic in CA, where I discovered I had celiac disease, depression, anxiety and more. Everything I was binging and purging on—gluten, dairy, and sugar—was making me sick and depleting my brain and body. Additionally, I learned about my candida issue, thyroid and adrenal dysfunction, and numerous nutrient deficiencies, particularly those affecting my brain's neurotransmitter production.

The outpatient clinic used targeted amino acid therapy to rebuild my severely depleted brain and within weeks, the binging and purging stopped, the depression and anxiety lifted, and I felt joy and hope for the first time. I had felt like I was crazy all those years with bulimia and came to find out…I wasn't crazy! My brain just needed to be nourished. I was finally able to react appropriately to stressors in my life and deal with what I needed to process in counseling. Amino Acid therapy literally saved my life and ignited my passion for nutritional therapy. For the past twenty-eight years now, I have implemented amino acid therapy, witnessing its transformative power in my life and my clients' lives. Miracles really do take place when the brain is nourished!

Amino Acid therapy can literally heal your brain from depression, anxiety and other mood and addiction challenges. When the brain is truly nourished, life stressors become more manageable, and then we can make the necessary diet and lifestyle changes to get to the root cause issues. A balanced brain allows us to view life positively and live vibrantly without mood medications and years of counseling.

You can't medicate away a nutrient deficiency…you have to fix it!

TIP: start your healing journey now

If you are struggling with anxiety, depression or addictions issues, consider using Amino Acid therapy to rebuild your brain and gain freedom in your life like never before. We are top down people and I firmly believe if we balance the brain with targeted amino acids in therapeutic doses, everything below the neck is easier to heal. I can help you with this!

Healing is possible, and it begins by nourishing your brain FIRST. Let's take back your brain and your life together.

* * *

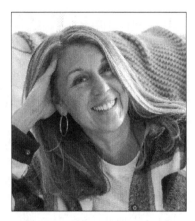

Learn More About Me

Holistic Health Specialist: As a functional nutritional therapist and neuro-nutrient specialist, I focus on brain health and emotional well-being.

Personal Triumphs: I've overcome my own health challenges, including cancer, celiac disease, bulimia, and depression, using advanced, holistic approaches.

Global Consultant: I work with clients from all over the world, both virtually and in person.

Empowerment Mission: My goal is to empower women (and a few men) to achieve optimal brain health and live free from anxiety, depression, and related health challenges.

Educational Advocate: Through coaching, classes, and workshops, I provide strategies and support to help you reclaim your health and live your best life.

To learn more about my journey and how I can help you reclaim your life from anxiety, depression, and addictions, visit https://www.lauriehammer.com/.

- Laurie Hammer, FNTP, NNTS
- Your favorite nutritional therapist
- https://www.facebook.com/takebackmybrain
- https://www.instagram.com/thecalmmomcommunity/
- https://www.youtube.com/channel/UCZw1GBitFZkaR8aSfbaOxeQ
- Podcast: https://www.lauriehammer.com/podcast

CHAPTER 7:

Cells that Shine at Any Age

By: Dr. Manuel Faria, DC, NMD, DACBN

What if there was a way to optimize your energy and vitality, optimize your health and healing and optimize your longevity health span, so that you don't just live longer but you actually live healthy longer? Wouldn't you want that more than anything? The greatest wealth you can have is your health. So take some time and invest it in knowledge that will give you the wisdom to apply these principles in your life.

People all over the world are looking for magic answers to their health and wellness solutions. Many times we forget the simple fact that all healing comes from the inside out. Health and healing are always the products of our own body's ability to maintain a state of balance amidst the internal and external forces and stressors that begin to create a state of dis-ease in the body. Dis-ease precludes disease. It is a state where the body is beginning to function in a less than optimal way.

We have an innate intelligence in the body that can bring the processes and mechanisms into play to heal itself and optimize function when the factors that interfere with this are identified and removed. I believe we all have the potential to live well past 100 years of age. I don't mean being old and riddled with chronic degenerative diseases and no memory of what we did in life. I mean cognitive and able to function in health and reflect on a life well lived. We will all die one day, I get that, but why not make a plan that puts into place an ability that will enable you to live healthy longer, and one day die healthy with a legacy left to your family and the people who knew your impact in the world.

So, what will it take to make the odds of this happening in your life possible? I have a saying, "If you treat your health today, you won't have to treat your disease tomorrow." The focus here will be on treating health not disease. Putting yourself always in the most optimal position of a body and mind that can heal itself given the right circumstances.

I have been in practice seeing thousands of patients over the last forty years. I not only teach these principles to my patients, but I have lived this way and applied these principles in my life on a daily basis. I want you to become the hero in your own health journey. I am now sixty-seven-years-old at the time of writing this. My biological age is younger than my physiological age and my rate or pace of aging is slower for every year lived as evidenced by testing. I still do high intensity functional fitness routines and I am actively learning new things and applying them in my life.

So what is the secret? Here we go. You need "cells that shine." There are over thirty trillion cells in the human body. Each one of those cells is a universe unto itself. Those cells make up your organs and your organs make up the systems of the body. Cells that shine are operating at their peak functional capacity to perform all the functions your body requires so that you can be optimally healthy. Cells have a lifespan. Old ones die off and new ones are created and the cycle goes on. Old cells that don't die when they should become senescent and begin to function in a way that hinders the body. You begin to have chronic inflammation that develops at the cellular level.

Think of your health as a sort of bucket. There is something called the bucket theory of disease. Imagine a bucket and you begin to fill it with water. There is a point when the bucket can't take anymore and it begins to overflow. That is when you begin to feel symptoms. It can take many years for that bucket to overflow. This cellular inflammation leads to dysfunctional mitochondria inside your cells.

So now what causes this cellular inflammation? The number one culprits are toxins. There are over 86,000 toxins and the number is growing everyday. They are in the food we eat, the air we breathe, the water we drink and so on. We don't live in a bubble, so we have to optimize our detox pathways at a cellular level daily and always.

Our cells also make up our GI system. We have thirty trillion cells in our body and those cells make up our digestive system. We have over thirty trillion organisms that live in our gut. This makes up the microbiome. It is a delicate ecosystem where more than seventy percent of our immune system resides. When out of balance, we can have overgrowth of harmful organisms, like parasites, viruses, fungus and bacteria.

All this leads to micronutrient deficiencies in the body and in the cells. So what I do on a daily basis is promote the "cells that shine" protocols in my own body and in my patients. Step one, promote cellular detox—lifestyle checkup and cellular formulas that heal and detox the cells. Step two, reduce harmful organisms in the gut. Step three, optimize and restore cellular functions with lifestyle protocols and specialized formulas that optimize health-span and longevity. We consult both in office and virtually.

* * *

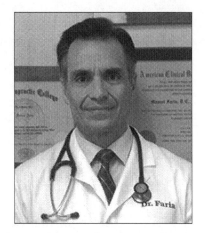

To learn more about what we do, contact **Dr. Manuel Faria, DC, NMD, DABCN**

Cellular Health Institute

195 South Westmonte Drive Suite 1116

Altamonte Springs, Florida 32714 Phone: 407-862-2287

www.healthecells.com

CHAPTER 8:

Where's My Energy?!?!

By: Sylvia J. Harral, MEd, NC, FBS

"STOP THE CAR!" Shouted the still, small voice in my gut as a wave of tiredness passed through my body. "AND WAKE YOURSELF UP!" My ego-head immediately countered my gut with logical reasoning: "You slept well last night." "You just finished hauling two loads of wood this morning." "You've eaten a good lunch; besides, you're going to be dancing in a few minutes, and that keeps you wide awake." My foot listened to my ego-head and kept the gas pedal at sixty MPH heading for a curve.

My heart and right lung were able to hang in long enough for the helicopter to arrive at the Fresno Community Hospital Trauma Center's Emergency Room 150 miles away. Sometime during thirteen hours in the Emergency Room, my heart and lung gave up; the left lung had collapsed. The extreme stillness I felt gripped my attention as I surrendered to it and fell asleep.

When I woke up, tubes were everywhere. Machines were monitoring everything my body did. One machine was down my throat breathing for me, and my stressed heart was still struggling through every beat.

That day, a scientist friend came to my bedside with a small bottle of herbal formula he had made in his medical-grade laboratory. He saw all the machines I was hooked up to and the blood pressure monitor that read 135/40. A small (actually HUGE) coincidence happened, and the herbal formula was put in my body. Minutes later, the diastolic blood pressure read 55; up fifteen points. "Got it!" He said, and left.

Five weeks later, I went home from the hospital. Six months later, I was dancing in the city park. Nine and a half years later, I'm still dancing, teaching, backpacking and writing this story.

Who was he, and what was in that bottle?

His name is Huu S. Tiêu. That part is simple, but to explain what was in the bottle will take a minute. It's something the Tiêu family has been researching for over 500 years. When his name is searched in Google Scholar, six peer reviewed journal articles appear. In them are written the scientific details of the new cellular-life-sparking technology he invented. I'll simplify the explanation like this:

When the sun goes down in the campground, we start wanting heat and light. We do three things in their proper order. 1) We gather the needed materials; pieces of wood, sticks, and kindling, 2) we strike the match, and 3) we enjoy heat and light enough to create lasting memories.

When it comes to a living cell, the same order exists. 1) Nutrients are gathered to form the cell and support life. 2) The spark of life causes the cell to become active and divide. 3) The cell performs its function.

As life happens, we may find our health slipping away and we're wishing for more energy. We don't often think about what's going on in our cells. They're too tiny to see and we're busy thinking about the big things in life. For example, we think more about having sex than about what those tiny cells will be doing for the next nine months or about how our life could change forever. We eat and drink what tastes good without thinking about the effects it will have on us in the long run. We take our health for granted. However, there are a few people who spend their entire lives thinking about the microscopic universe we don't see. They figure out how things happen, calculate the details and write the equations for things like cellular functions.

Albert Einstein thought about the energy production; the third stage. He did not give us a practical application of $E=MC2$, because it's everywhere around us. The E stands for energy. $E=MC2$ is seen in the function of a cell, a firecracker, the atom bomb (YIKES! A little too much heat and light), or a supernova (which would make the atom bomb look like a firecracker). Einstein won a Nobel Prize for his equation in 1921.

Erin Schrödinger figured out the calculations and equation for the first stage; the gathering of nutrients needed to form a cell and keep it functioning. He won the Nobel Prize in 1933. He couldn't provide a practical application for his equation, but he wrote a book about it called, *What is Life?* His equation is too long and complicated to be included here, but a part of it looks like this: $\Psi(x, t) = Aei(kx - \omega t)$.

Scientists knew the spark was there but were unable to work out the calculations and equation to explain the details of its existence. It took a third scientist with a thorough enough understanding and imagination to finally get all the calculations right.

Huu S. Tiêu figured out the equation for the spark of life sixty years after Schrodinger won his Nobel Prize. The Tiêu Equation is $E=HI\Psi T/P$, however, it was kept a secret for thirty years. Huu wanted to develop its practical application first. The Tiêu Equation Technology supports cellular life well enough to relieve mankind's suffering from disease; his family's dream for over 500 years.

Using his extensive knowledge of herbs and cellular functions, he fermented plants for two years. This causes the atoms in the molecular structures to be released. The atoms are then recombined into new molecular protein structures when passed through the "technology tube" in his lab. The new protein structures have quick, positive effects on cellular function, because they complete all three equations in each living cell.

41

The practical application is a liquid that can be administered easily. It can be dropped under the tongue for a couple minutes (and it tastes terrible by the way). It can be dropped into an empty capsule and swallowed without tasting it, or put through a feeding tube like it was given to me. (My favorite way to swallow it is with a bite of food.)

The Tiêu Equation Technology (TET) is what was in the bottle. That's what caused my blood pressure to change for the better so quickly. That's what gave my cells the needed energy to heal.

The Journal of Natural Science > Vol.15 No.3, March 2023, lists a few facts about the Tiêu Equation Technology.

Its impressive benefits are measured through the consistent improvement in blood reports and other diagnostic tests. The TET provides a wave function which moves nutrient particles through the blood-brain-barrier and cell walls with temperature producing energy. This streamlines the cell's return to thriving health and keeps it functioning in the top-of-its-game.

Our cells are built to thrive but designed to survive. When either the variety or supply of nutrients diminishes, the cells switch from thriving to survival mode. In survival mode, they continue to function as best they can on nutrients they borrow from each other. Many cells survive a long-time off loans-from-the-bones. (Poor bones!)

The TET comes with a hefty supply of rare nutrients, plus it's a one-of-a-kind delivery system for all nutrients. Its quantum tunneling action brings nutrients right through the cell wall without damaging the nutrient or the wall. When the long-awaited nutrients arrive, cells rejoice, kick out toxins, and return to normal function. Healing energy, anyone?

The TET eases suffering from serious, life-threatening diseases or conditions, because it makes inflammation work for the body instead of against it. Inflammation is the first step in the healing process. Inflammation brings swelling, heat, redness, pain, and reduced mobility. The swelling brings nutrients and immune cells to the healing site. The heat makes the immune cells work faster and more efficiently. The redness is the result of increased circulation, and temperature. Pain lets us know there's work in progress and nutrients are needed to support the healing process. Reduced mobility is necessary to avoid further injury. The TET's delivery system expedites healing by flooding the cells with nutrients. As healing progresses, the need for inflammation goes away and so does the swelling and redness. We love it when mobility is restored without the pain.

When people seek their return to health, their journey to success is enhanced by the addition of the Tiêu Equation Technology. It doesn't replace the need for all dietary supplements, it just makes them work better. This reduces the need for as many supplements and speeds up the results. There are no side effects or contraindications with medications. I've watched the effects of thousands of servings in and on the bodies of people and animals. Everyone is unique and special. Health is expensive, but how many diseases can we afford.

I start my clients with the Tiêu Equation Technology along with the powerful supplements and protocols we use in our bloodwork consultations and programs. The TET puts the body on its Natural Healing Pathway with the first drop. Then we learn to follow that pathway to health. That takes energy!

Feel free to contact me at familyhelm@hotmail.com.

* * *

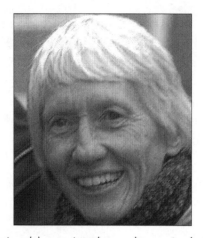

Sylvia is a natural-born teacher who puts her lessons into analogies to help her students grasp the lessons more completely. From the first grade up, she mentally rehearsed being a teacher. She completed her Licensed Practical Nurse's training at Walla Walla Community College then received her bachelor's degree from Walla Walla University. She taught Physical Education at the college level then finished her master's degree at Utah State University. Today, she focuses her attention on teaching people to take charge of their health at the cellular level, where it counts the most. She authored the *Body-Languages & Body-Money Manual* which was used as a textbook in her college health course for fifteen years. Her love of nature, children, and backpacking culminated in the *Teddy Bear Adventure Series* of books for children. Sylvia is the *Public Relations & Event Organizer* for The *Altruistic United Humanity Association*, a 501 (c) (3), charitable organization that handles donations for Medical Treatment and Medical Research. She also developed the *Body And Soul & Earth (BASE) Restoration* treatment program where she reads clients bloodwork and recommends cutting edge practitioner-only lines of dietary supplements along with the Tiêu Equation Technology products from *Golden Sunrise Nutraceutical*.

CHAPTER 9:

Do You Need To Take Out The Trash?

By: Beth Krause, CFNLP, CNC, MA

Have you ever had a time in your life where you had a lot of trash that seemed to pile up and you didn't know what you were going to do to get rid of it? Translate that to your health. Do you have health conditions that seem to keep piling up and you can not find answers for them?

Finding ways to navigate your health is like taking out the trash. You must have a system in place in order to find a method not to overwhelm you. When I look at helping my clients with their complex health issues we start from the beginning.

We focus on the five pillars of health starting with mindset. Many in the Functional Health space would consider this the last pillar, but quite frankly, I feel that this is the very foundation of our existence and therefore needs to be where we begin. I am a faith-based provider; therefore, we are going to take a minute to look at your trash from a spiritual perspective.

You must be able to create a sense of safety, a sense of relaxation, a place for reflection, and a connection through prayer. We must be able to clear the negative thinking and the societal pressures that have already been placed in the spaces in our mind in order to overcome the negativity that we have already taken on so that we are able to move forward in our healing journey. The mind is a very powerful tool and can be used against us if we allow it, however, we can also use it to our benefit by giving ourselves gratitude affirmations every single day. Let's face it, some of us will need to be reminded of these affirmations by posting post-it notes all over. We were created by a Creator to have a connection, to be relational beings. To give up that spiritual baggage we have been carrying around, we need to allow our Creator to take it from us.

While I had one of my clients in my clinic, I was visiting with them while working on them and I could feel that there was a sticking point during the appointment. I said, "I have to stay right here for a moment, there is something going on here and it feels like there is some kind of blockage." I asked them, "Do you have something going on that you haven't shared with me recently or you would like to share with me right now? If not, that is ok too, but it feels like it may be emotional, it feels like whatever it is, it is building up and not releasing." Suddenly the floodgates of emotions started to flow out of my client. There was definitely an emotional, spiritual, and family issue that had happened since our last time together. They continued to pour out what had been happening and the more they shared, the more the blockage started to release. The more the blockage released, the deeper I was able to go with our therapy. When our session was finished and they were preparing to leave, they said, "I feel like an emotional and physical noodle, but I really needed to let all that go! Thank you so much, I didn't know I had stored all of that up." Are you holding on to something that you need to let go?

What you are holding onto right now is like piling up the trash. Take a deep reflective look to see what it is that you could do today to let something go. Do you have unresolved conflict, someone you need to forgive, anger that hasn't been dealt with, a wrong that needs to be corrected. All these things can be overcome. It just takes a moment of your time. Stepping out of your comfort zone. A change in your mindset. Your mind is a powerful tool. Choose to use it or partner with someone that will help you obtain the necessary tools to move forward and help you start to eliminate the trash in your life.

We also store unnecessary trash in our gut. When we are not digesting properly, we hold onto so much sludge. We do not absorb the necessary nutrients, we hold on to toxins because we are not eliminating properly. This may lead to leaky gut/leaky brain causing several ongoing health issues that become uncomfortable. These conditions may look like: chronic constipation, chronic diarrhea, nausea, indigestion, reflux, headaches, brain fog, fatigue, and inflammation. Sound familiar? Once detoxification is properly nurtured and supported with proper nutritive supplements and herbs, the gut can start the healing process.

Getting proper nutrition requires first knowing your body's needs and then giving your body the food and supplements that will improve your health. Now, I realize that everyone has a different school of thought on what nutritional guidelines to follow. Functional medicine recognizes that nutritional choices must be based on what each individual needs and that may vary significantly from person to person. This is where finding out what our clients' yes or no lists are and why they have chosen those foods. This list may have ties to their emotional/spiritual mindset as well. Essentially, everyone should focus on eating a rainbow of whole foods.

While knowing and starting to understand how your body works, we are barely scratching the surface. You are probably wanting to know what you can do right now, right?

Some tips that I suggest to my clients when they are looking for emotional grounding and safety to be able to release deep emotions is to begin with deep breathing. This type of breathing is a deep and reflective breathing technique. You feel this breath deep in the base of your lungs and full in your diaphragm. Breathe completely out and deep for as long as you can and then take that deep inhale all the way to the tippy top of your head, but keeping your shoulders relaxed. Repeat this three times.

I also recommend using a castor oil pack over your abdomen at night. This can help with gut inflammation, pain, detox, stress and emotional release.

I have a morning routine that you are able to take advantage of today!

https://www.graceanatomyfunctionalhealth.com/morningroutine

✳ ✳ ✳

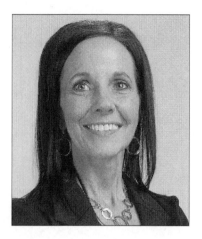

My name is **Beth Krause**, CFNLP, CNC, MA, Certified Functional Bloodwork Specialist, and Certified Pain Relief Therapist. I am a certified Functional Health and Nutrition Practitioner that empowers clients through education and guidance while supporting them in their pursuit of wellness. I am the bridge for my clients as an advocate for their health. My goal is to help give you the tools that you can utilize in everyday life that will help serve you the best.

I am a child of God, wife, mother and "Oma" to twelve (soon to be thirteen) grand-babies. I love the outdoors, horses, dogs and chickens. Trail riding, gardening, hiking, and spending time with my family are some of my favorite things to do.

I am happy to know that you are here, let's connect by email: hello@graceanatomyfunctionalhealth.com or visit my website @ https://www.graceanatomyfunctionalhealth.com/

CHAPTER 10:

The Big C

By: Ally Harmon

The Big C. Cancer. That horrifying six letter word that no one ever wants to hear. Yet, in today's American culture, with statistics showing one out of every two people will develop cancer at some point during their lifetime, it seems inescapable. One must wonder, what has changed in the last sixty years to make those statistics more than double? Why are we a society leading the charts not only in cancer, but also in inflammation, autoimmune disorders, heart disease, and psychiatric illness? What do other cultures know that we do not?

The fact is, like sheep without a shepherd, we have lost our way. We have lost touch with our connection to the old teachings of living in a symbiotic relationship with our environment and the food we eat. We have lost confidence in our innate ability to use the gifts that God has given us by way of the earth. Everything we need is here at our fingertips. We do not typically need fancy labs and expensive, designer drugs. We do not need to be poked and prodded like lab rats and given toxic potions that make our hair fall out, our skin fall off, and fractionate our quality of life. What we do need is a little faith in our body's own innate ability to heal, when given the proper tools and support.

Let us take a look at a patient whose primary care physician called "the walking medical nightmare." She struggled with autoimmune disorders, frequent seizures, chronic fatigue, chronic pain, ADHD and depression. She was in and out of hospitals with a myriad of issues, and no one could ever figure out what was wrong. Every test came back normal. Some doctors would become frustrated and tell the girl, "This is a somatic issue," or, "it's all in your head." At the age of thirty-seven, the girl was in a go-karting accident and needed a CT scan. The emergency room physician walked in and said, "The ribs are only bruised, but there is a mass in the chest." The girl laughed it off, stating, "No one in the family has ever had cancer, so it couldn't possibly be that." A couple months later she reluctantly got some follow-up scans. The results showed a grade three tumor in the breast, and she was diagnosed with a rare and aggressive form of breast cancer known as Triple Negative Breast Cancer. The prognosis was grim. The treatments available were few. The fear was high. That girl was me.

Getting diagnosed with cancer places one onto an assembly line of sorts, full of medical oncologists, radiation oncologists, surgical oncologists, plastic surgeons, genetic testing specialists, insurance specialists, nurses and counselors. When you sit before these specialists, whom you think hold all the answers, and therefore, the keys to whether you get to live or not, it is hard *not* to see them as omnipotent beings, and trust anything and everything that comes from their mouths. They expect this. They expect you to do exactly as they suggest. And why wouldn't you? They have your best interest at heart, right?

When it comes to a cancer diagnosis, western medicine gives three options: cut it out, drown it in chemo or radiate it. And if those do not work, then become a guinea pig in a research trial where you may or may not be given any real chance at survival with an experimental new drug (no one is told whether or not they get the real thing or the placebo).

My medical oncologist told me that I needed a strong course of chemo with three different chemo drugs if I wanted any real chance at making it to a two-year survival, following surgery and eight weeks of radiation. When I asked how, statistically speaking, would doing this chemo raise my chances of survival versus not doing it at all, her response was "six percent." For clarification, I would be receiving a chemo course so strong that it kills nearly 25% of people and leaves 60-70% of those who survive with such brain damage that they cannot put a coherent sentence together six months post-treatment...all for a 6% chance that I might survive two years.

I was in graduate school at the time and was unwilling to give up my brain. If chemotherapy only extends life, on average, by an extra two weeks, and there was only a six percent chance that it would even do that, I would rather have quality over quantity. I walked away knowing that chemo would kill me, and I wanted to live. There had to be another way.

I intuitively knew that I needed to build up my immune system, not tear it down. I found doctors out of Germany and began learning their treatment protocols. They had a natural substance with extensive research showing it to be five times more effective than chemo. I quickly put together a team and developed a naturopathic treatment protocol. We began importing the injectables from Germany. I met with a cancer nutritionist, and we put together a special diet to help support the body so it could fight the cancer optimally: a modified, medical ketogenic diet. Weekly high dose vitamin C infusions to increase apoptosis. Daily infrared sauna treatments. Specialty supplements to regulate blood sugars, deplete blood supply to the cancer cells, and support the liver for breaking down dying cancer cells. Coffee enemas to flush the bile from the liver carrying the cancer cells and other wastes. Juicing. Gentle exercise. Affirmations. Joy. Cleaning out toxic relationships. And a whole heck of a lot of prayer. I was not a religious person at the time, but I did pray, "God, if you let me survive this, I promise to spend the rest of my life helping others learn what I have learned about cancer and teaching them that they can overcome this." I began to see cancer differently. It was no longer the curse I first thought it was; I came to see it as a gift. That was ten years ago. And I am still cancer free.

Everyone has to walk their own path after a cancer diagnosis, but it is not a path that has to be walked alone. You are not stuck or trapped or doomed. You DO have choices. You DO have options. You get to decide how you want to feel moving through your journey and what you want that journey to look like. YOU are in the driver's seat.

It is God's calling and my life's mission to help those who want to fight and survive a cancer diagnosis, and to do it whilst promoting quality of life. As women, we have a tendency to hold our traumas in our breast tissue. When left untreated, this trauma turns to inflammation, and inflammation can turn into cancer. It takes time, patience, and dedication to overcome, as the dis-ease did not occur overnight. Through mind-body-spirit work, healing is possible.

* * *

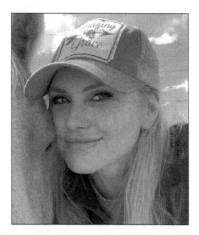

Ally Harmon lives in Arvada, Colorado, where she runs Two Wolves Healing Sanctuary on a small horse farm. She worked as an equine-facilitated psychotherapist for children and ex-military prior to her cancer diagnosis. After healing, she earned degrees in Integrative Health Practices and Nursing, along with certifications in Frequency Specific Microcurrent, Functional Blood Analysis, Integrative Somatic Trauma Therapy, Energy Medicine, Usui and Holy Fire Reiki master/teacher, Ayurvedic breathwork, holistic nutrition, and Healing Touch-RN. She is currently working towards her doctorate and PhD in Integrative Medicine, while seeing patients in private and group settings. She can be reached by emailing Lharmon@regis.edu

CHAPTER 11

Insulin Resistance: America's Silent Epidemic

By: Sybil Coburn

Always hungry? Can't lose weight and struggle to have enough energy to get through your day? Does this sound like you? How about high triglycerides, low HDL (good) cholesterol and blood pressure that keeps creeping up? If the pounds keep packing on and the scale won't budge no matter what you do, there is a good chance you could have insulin resistance. Are you thinking, "Surely not! My doctor has never mentioned this to me." Well, that's because they are not looking for it. The signs are there, and the proof is in your "normal" blood work, but more often than not, the necessary tests are not run.

Type II Diabetes is the result of insulin resistance that is not diagnosed or treated properly. The condition is typically diagnosed with elevated glucose and Hemoglobin A1c. It can take up to ten years of insulin resistance before Type II diabetes is diagnosed. By the time these lab tests become out of range, the damage of insulin resistance has wreaked havoc on the body.

Insulin resistance leads to hyperglycemia, hypertension, dyslipidemia, hyperuricemia, elevated inflammatory markers, endothelial dysfunction and a prothrombic state. What does all that mean? Prolonged elevated insulin results in Type II diabetes, cardiovascular disease, gout, systemic inflammation, fatty liver and blood clots. But wait, isn't the treatment for Type II Diabetes insulin injections? Yes, it is. But treatment of diabetes with insulin does not resolve the underlying insulin resistance. That is why diabetics tend to gain weight, have a high risk of cardiovascular disease, chronic inflammation and the need for more and more insulin as time goes on.

Insulin acts like a key to unlock the receptor(lock) on the cell allowing glucose to enter. With prolonged elevated insulin exposure, the cells decrease the number of receptors (locks) that the key fits into, resulting in too much glucose in the blood. The body responds by producing more insulin which in turn causes the cells to remove more receptors (locks) from the cell surface causing a vicious cycle. This cycle leads to obesity, inflammation and diabetes. This is a cycle I know all too well, as I have personal experience with insulin resistance.

I knew I was headed down the path to diabetes when my weight was well over 200 lbs. I was obese, had chronic fatigue, debilitating asthma, constipation, brain fog, joint pain, anxiety, depression, hot flashes, mood swings, sleep disturbances and could not lose weight. I had tried cutting calories and exercising which left me in bed exhausted and in pain. Nothing seemed to work, and I was feeling desperate. I knew going through menopause feeling like this would be unbearable.

Being a chiropractic doctor, I have in depth knowledge of biochemical pathways of the body and familiarity with supplements to support those pathways. However, the calories in/calories out approach was not working for me the way it once had when I was younger. That is because I had become insulin resistant. I had to dive into the research to discover how to break the vicious cycle of insulin resistance. Through implementing these new strategies and techniques I was able to lose sixty pounds, eliminate the hot flashes, brain fog and other symptoms I was suffering from.

Now I have my life back! Not only am I a healthy weight again, my asthma has all but disappeared. I have plenty of energy to get through my day and look forward to exercising. My hormones have regulated, and I no longer have constant food cravings or mood swings. I did this by addressing the insulin resistance. That was the missing link. The insulin resistance was why my prior efforts were not working. Through this process I have developed a program to help others break the cycle of insulin resistance and overcome their unique health challenges as well.

Breaking the cycle of insulin resistance can seem impossible unless you have a specific road map to follow. I have developed such a road map and specialize in helping people return to health. I am a functional blood work specialist, so I customize every program based on an individual's unique presentation and blood work. A few of the tests I look at when addressing insulin resistance are fasting insulin and Vitamin D.

Insufficient levels of Vitamin D decrease the number of insulin receptors (locks) on the membrane of our cells contributing to insulin resistance. Optimal Vitamin D level is 80 to 100 ng/ml. For more information on how to reverse insulin resistance, non-alcoholic fatty liver disease or to find out more about the programs I offer, contact me at www.DrSybilNutrition.com.

* * *

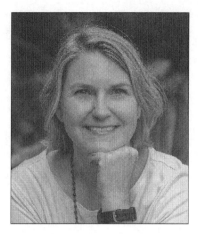

Dr. Sybil Coburn

Chiropractor and Metabolic Health Specialist

Hello! I'm Dr. Sybil Coburn, and I'm passionate about helping people overcome insulin resistance, diabetes, pre-diabetes, fatty liver, and cholesterol challenges naturally. By integrating tailored nutrition plans, lifestyle changes, and holistic strategies, I empower individuals to reclaim their health and vitality.

I have created a twelve-week program called "Take Back Your Life" to coach people with diabetes on how to improve their health & lower A1c. You can sign up for this course today at www. DrSybilNutrition.com

Join me on this journey toward better metabolic health by connecting with me on social media or through my website:

https://www.facebook.com/sybil.coburn

https://www.instagram.com/sybilcoburn/

www.DrSybilNutrition.com

CHAPTER 12:

How Your Thyroid Works... Simplified

By: Dr. Barbara Layne Jennings

My hair was falling out by the handful. I couldn't get off the sofa to play with my kids, my hands shook, my heart skipped beats. I had restless legs, couldn't sleep and a troublesome cough.

"I've never been really sick before. How did I get so sick?" I asked my endocrinologist. His answer was completely unsatisfactory: "We don't know. Some people just do. So don't exercise because your heart could stop, and make your treatment choice soon."

He had just diagnosed me with Toxic Multinodular Goiter, an "incurable" autoimmune hyperthyroid condition and my choice was between surgery to remove my thyroid OR drinking radioactive iodine to kill my thyroid. Both extreme options would leave me dependent on medication for the rest of my life. At age twenty-eight I didn't want that!

I knew nothing about my thyroid or why I got sick, but my instincts told me there had to be a better option, one that would help me actually HEAL MY BODY.

A chiropractor helped me achieve "the impossible"—a natural recovery! With diet changes, natural tools & adjustments to relieve stress, in six months my symptoms were gone. My hair and my energy were coming back, and I could be a mom again! This was in 1999; I never had the surgery or radioactive iodine and I'm still in excellent health.

I learned three important things; if I remove things that interfere with the way my body works, it can start working again. There was a reason I got sick, and my body can heal!

This inspired me to become a doctor to help others who suffer from thyroid problems. It's SO common, and it's often unnecessary to have surgery or destructive treatments.

Here's my "Superman analogy" to help explain how the thyroid works with so many parts of your body. It includes Clark Kent, Superman, a phone booth, & kryptonite:

The thyroid makes two main hormones, T4 and T3. T4 is like Clark Kent, the inactive hormone. T3 is like Superman, the active hormone that makes things happen.

The thyroid makes 93% Clark Kent (T4), and only 7% Superman (T3). This is actually a safety measure to ensure your cells don't get dangerously over-stimulated.

So all these Clark Kent T4s must convert into Superman T3s to get your metabolism working right. And where does Clark Kent change into Superman? The phone booth…

In this analogy, the phone booth is your liver. But an unhealthy liver is not able to efficiently convert T4 (Clark Kent) into T3 (Superman). Thus liver function is a crucial factor, especially with low thyroid symptoms, yet it is often overlooked by doctors.

After the liver conversion, T3 is carried in the blood to its receptors on every cell. Those receptors must be open and able to connect, not blocked by toxins and inflammation.

T3 hormone is special; it stimulates every single cell to do its job. This is a critical part of your metabolism. Cells need just the right amount of T3 hormone. Too little and the cell will be slow and tired, too much and they will be over-stimulated and over-active. Both cause symptoms and can be dangerous if severe.

Consider your brain and heart, neither should be under-stimulated and slow, as that can feel like depression, anxiety, brain fog, fatigue, hair loss and irregular heart rhythm. Over-stimulation can feel like insomnia, hyperactivity or fatigue, hair loss and irregular heart rhythm.

Your body constantly communicates with your brain about whether it is receiving the right amount of T3 stimulation. Your brain (pituitary gland) responds with TSH (thyroid stimulating hormone), which is the gas pedal to your thyroid. More gas (a higher TSH) = body needs more stimulation. Less gas (a lower TSH) = body wants less stimulation.

Kryptonite are the toxins that block T3 receptors, and also iodine receptors in the thyroid gland: fluoride, chlorine, bromine. Avoid these and detox to remove them!

The number 3 or 4 in T3 & T4 tell you the # of molecules of iodine in T3 & T4. So without iodine, you cannot make T3 or T4 so iodine is essential for your thyroid, your metabolism & overall health. (*But don't start supplementing iodine without a health practitioner who knows how to do this safely!)

Actions you can take now to support your body towards natural healing:

1. A diet change is a must: avoid gluten, soy, dairy, & often corn. It may seem hard at first, but the payoff of feeling great is well worth it!

2. Get tested to find out if you have autoimmune antibodies. See a complete thyroid panel here https://drbarbarajennings. com/thyroid-health/

3. Improve liver function with detox, like this https://detox. drbarbarajennings.com

* * *

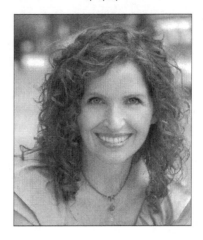

Dr. Jennings helps people all over North America with individual and group programs:

www.DrBarbaraJennings.com &

https://www.facebook.com/HealthSummit/

CHAPTER 13:

The Night That Changed Everything: From Desperation to Discovery

By: Amy Dilena, DC, ACN, FDNP and
Functional Bloodwork Specialist

It was around midnight, so we knew the routine. I go get my son, and my husband grabs the blanket. We meet in the garage with the door open so he can breathe in the cool, damp, foggy air. Sometimes we would drive around with the windows down at 1 a.m., and if it was really bad, we would end up in the ER. That only happened a couple of times when they would give him a steroid injection to help reduce the swelling. My son was four years old, and this wasn't our first time, unfortunately. He had what the doctors called croup. I had it as a little girl, and the way it was described to us was a viral infection that causes swelling of the throat. As he grows and his airway becomes bigger, he will grow out of it. According to the doctors, age five was the magic number when we could put this "routine" behind us. The scariest part to me was that it would occur out of the blue.

One of the earlier episodes happened while my parents were watching the boys, and my husband and I were going out of town for the weekend. My son was totally fine when we left that afternoon. By the time we were in the taxi on our way to the hotel after a one-hour plane ride, we got the call that they were in the ER. We were on the next plane home.

This particular night started out as it typically did. I would hear the distinctive coughing and go in to get him, but as I went to pick up my baby boy, something was different. The gasp for air was urgent, he was quieter, his lips were blue, and his eyes looked scared. I shouted to my husband to call 9-1-1 and rushed my baby out the front door to the cool air. The paramedics arrived so fast. They got the swelling down right away, and he could breathe again.

I vowed at that moment we weren't going to just 'live like this' until he grew out of it. We needed answers NOW. After multiple visits with his pediatrician, the best solution was to keep an EpiPen on hand. My parents and siblings lived in a more rural area about thirty minutes from us, with no cell phone range, and it would take paramedics fifteen minutes to arrive in an emergency. The pediatrician recommended we either don't leave city limits or always carry the EpiPen.

This began my quest for "real answers." As a chiropractor, I understood the nervous system and the innate intelligence, but I was struggling to understand what was really happening in his body. As he "grew" out of croup, he developed severe eczema. It covered his elbows and knees and the cheeks on his face.

In college, I suffered from anxiety and panic attacks. However, I was never actually told that was what it was; I figured it out on my own. When the medical route ruled out a heart attack, and I was told everything in my labs was normal and I must be suffering from depression, I was prescribed Prozac and Xanax. That is when I took matters into my own hands and refused to live a life in fear.

Running into the same dead end with my son's health, I decided to do the same, take matters into our own hands. We ran food sensitivity testing. The results were very difficult to enforce. What do you feed a five-year-old when the list of foods he was sensitive to were the main staples he ate and included things such as yeast, eggs, pepper, and tomatoes—all ingredients in many food dishes? I tried, but it was nearly impossible. I refused to give up. I knew there was an answer. But, the real answer I wanted to find was WHY did he have food sensitivities in the first place? If we could answer that question, we could find the answer to his healing.

My own health challenges led me to learn and understand HOW the body works and the vital key component—nutrition. The vitamins, minerals, and the body's ability to absorb and assimilate these nutrients, how this was the foundation to healing. But how do we know if we are getting the right or wrong nutrition? There are a bazillion diets out there: keto, paleo, eat more protein, eat more fat, intermittent fast, etc. So how do we know what our individual body needs?

This is when I learned about functional labs. Reading labs through a functional lens helps us find clues as to how our body is functioning. And from those clues, we are able to adapt lifestyle and dietary habits to heal and improve function. Yes, my son had sensitivities to a ton of very healthy foods, but his body was unable to digest, process, and absorb them properly. That was the missing link! Not the need for an EpiPen or to limit our distance of travel.

The same went for me. My panic and anxiety weren't something I was born with; it developed after a handful of years of poor dietary habits and high levels of stress, burning the candle at both ends while in graduate school.

By looking at my "normal" labs through a functional lens, I was able to see I had an underlying infection, very low Vitamin D and low TSH. My immune system was weakened, and my liver and gut health were poor. I wasn't able to absorb my nutrients properly. The symptoms presented as neck pain, radiating into my arms, anxiety, panic attacks, brain fog, not to mention frustration and feelings of hopelessness. This all changed when I found the clues and took action to heal.

The same went for my son. He is now a healthy adult with no food sensitivities and no signs of eczema. If you have suffered with unexplained health challenges or chronic health issues and have been told, all your labs look "normal," the same can be true for you, too!

If you are interested in learning what your "normal" labs mean and how the clues from reading them from a functional perspective can provide answers to your chronic health issues, I'd be honored to help you! Please visit my website at www.nutritionforhealth.net to learn more about how you can find the solutions and answers to your health challenges.

* * *

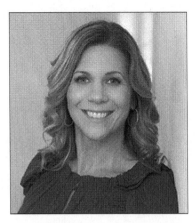

Amy Dilena, DC, ACN, FDNP and Functional Bloodwork Specialist

With over twenty years of experience in the natural holistic health care field, I have honed my expertise to help people in their health journey. As a Chiropractor, Functional Blood Work specialist and a certified practitioner in Functional Diagnostic Nutrition and Applied Clinical Nutrition, my focus has always been on addressing the whole person.

My approach is unique. I specialize in utilizing everyday "normal" routine laboratory tests as a tool to uncover hidden imbalances in the body. By interpreting these tests through the lens of functional medicine, I am able to identify and address underlying issues that often go unnoticed in standard medical evaluations.

I believe that the path to healing lies in both nutrition and lifestyle habits. My goal is to help people heal naturally, using their body's own intelligence and capabilities. Through personalized nutrition and lifestyle adjustments, I guide my patients towards optimal health, enabling them to lead fulfilling and vibrant lives.

My passion lies in helping others achieve their health goals. My mission is to empower each individual with the knowledge and resources to take control of their health. And my obsession? Optimal health, not just as a concept, but as a practical, achievable state of being for everyone I work with.

Join me in this journey towards holistic health and wellness. Together, we can unlock the secrets your body holds and harness them for a healthier, happier you.

CHAPTER 14:

Releasing Weight: A Journey to Health and Healing

By: Christina Smith BSN, RN, Certified Life Coach, Functional Blood Work Specialist

Struggling with weight issues can be incredibly challenging, both physically and emotionally. For years, I believed my weight problems were entirely my fault. While I had some bad habits, especially with sugar, the full story was much more complex.

My Struggle with Weight

After having two babies, I could never return to my pre-pregnancy weight, no matter how hard I exercised or followed the latest fad diets. This was incredibly discouraging. My doctors offered very little help & repeatedly told me to exercise more and eat less. This advice took a severe toll on my psyche, leaving me feeling depressed, guilty, ashamed and a failure.

Challenges with the Medical System

In addition to my weight issues, I suffered from chronic migraines, hypothyroidism, joint pain, fatigue and digestive problems. All of the stress from the unresolved issues changed the hypothyroidism into Hashimoto's. Each symptom led to a new diagnosis and more medications. I felt trapped in a medical system that wasn't helping & despite my doctor's assurances that my lab results were normal, I continued to struggle.

Finding Functional Medicine

Eventually, I reached nearly 300 pounds and felt utterly defeated. Determined to find answers, I turned to functional medicine. To my surprise, the solutions were hidden in my "normal" blood work. Here are a few tips for those who have struggled with weight and feel let down by the medical system. There is hope and your body can heal. I promise!

Proper Blood Work Analysis

Get your blood work analyzed properly for hidden infections or imbalances that may be preventing weight release. Find a trained functional blood work specialist who can provide answers for optimal living.

Have you ever had your doctor tell you your labs are normal, yet you still feel like something is wrong? I relate to this because it happened to me. I lived with "normal" labs for years before learning I had underlying infections that could be treated naturally without medication. The healthcare system often focuses on diagnosing and managing symptoms rather than finding the root cause.

The Importance of a Coach

Get a coach to help you on your journey. Find someone who has walked a similar path and can offer guidance and support. If you're like me, you've tried countless exercise and diet programs only to be disappointed. Years of failure had me believing it was impossible to release weight, especially with an autoimmune disease.

My coach helped me change my mindset, and offered real sustainable solutions that I chose to believe would finally work. And when that shift happened, the weight finally released. With the right guidance, weight is no longer an issue. In fact, my body has released over 120 pounds. A coach can teach you sustainable lifestyle changes that include movement, great food and releasing mind blocks that keep you stuck.

Changing Your Mindset

Change your mindset from "losing" weight to "releasing" weight. This shift can help your brain feel safer and more willing to let go of the extra pounds. The human brain is designed to keep us safe and comfortable. It perceives loss as a threat, which triggers a fight-or-flight response. Even if the extra weight is unhealthy, the brain sees it as familiar and safe which keeps us feeling stuck in a stress response. That response is great if truly in danger, but does not serve us well when trying to release weight.

Have a conversation with yourself. Tell your brain, "I am safe and I can easily release weight" or "releasing weight is easy for us." Be kind to yourself, just as you would be to your best friend. For those days that are really tough, have a pep talk ready to offer yourself comfort. Have your own back so to speak.

What Can You Do Right Now to Start Feeling Better?

Maybe you don't have as much weight to release as I did. Maybe you just have some pesky pounds hanging around that won't go away no matter what you do. Maybe you just don't feel quite right and need some answers. Reach out to me, we can work together to find solutions that are right for you.

If weight is an issue for you, start with simple things like drinking more water and some gentle movement like stretching or a stroll around the block. These two simple things can have a huge impact on how you feel right now. Don't forget to reach out to me! And more importantly, be kind to yourself. Understand that it's easy to fall into a model of being sick and once you're there you need some help changing that model. I wholeheartedly believe that's why I walked the path I did, so that I could find & help someone just like YOU! I understand all the negative feelings that come with feeling misunderstood. Let's get out of merely surviving and start thriving!

73

✶ ✶ ✶

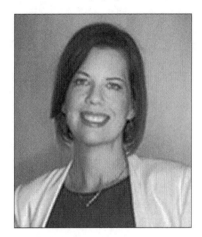

Christina Smith BSN, RN, Certified Life Coach, Functional Blood Work Specialist and international best-seller with her co-authored book *Healing Beyond the Diagnosis, Volume 2*

As a person that has released over 120 pounds using principles of functional medicine, I am an expert in how to heal the body and mind without intense exercise and fad diets. I have learned how to balance the body and mind to release weight. My ultimate goal is to help people heal their minds and their bodies to live life to their fullest potential. After all, life is so much sweeter when the mind and body are aligned!

On a personal note, together my husband and I raised two phenomenal sons while he served as an active-duty military member in the U.S. Navy. We also have a beautiful daughter-in-law and grandson. Now that we are empty nesters, we have new adventures in travel. Some of my favorite things to do are to assemble puzzles, play with my grandson and spend time with my family along with several dogs and cats that bring me great comfort!

You can reach me at:Facebook: Christina Smith

Email: thatfunctionalcoach@gmail.com

Website: thatfunctionalcoach.com

CHAPTER 15:

The Bloodwork Markers That May Explain Why You Keep Losing Energy, Stamina & Momentum In Your Career & Life

By: Julie Richard, FNS-BC, FMS, CNAS, CNS

Imagine waking up every morning feeling like you've only slept for an hour, even though you've had a full night's rest. Imagine going to your high stress job every day knowing that by noon you will be running fever with body aches and chills yet expected to perform at the high level your career demands. Imagine what would happen if your career, or even your life, got shifted off course. What if the answer lies in your bloodwork, specifically in the markers your doctor might be overlooking?

According to a 2020 McKinsey report, approximately one-in-four women consider downshifting their career or leaving the workforce entirely due to various health-related issues. Another survey conducted by Public Health England suggested that up to 30% of women experienced severe health symptoms that affected their ability to work leading to career and job instability. Lastly, 80% of the autoimmune population worldwide are, you guessed it, women.

In the summer of 2016, I became one of those statistics. My career as a high level chemical engineer in management shifted when my body began "shutting down" with no explanation. My job performance slipped and I found myself on "long term disability" due to my inability to work consistently. Doctor after doctor gave me few answers and little explanation as to what was happening. I wish I could tell you how many times I heard, "You are young. You are healthy. You shouldn't be having this pain," and "Your labs are pretty normal. There's nothing wrong." The situations I asked you to imagine yourself in is what I dealt with daily for many, many months. After several years, many doctors, many tests and scans, tons of money and a very major surgery, I finally had a list of autoimmune disorders that I could label myself with.

By nature, I am an annoyingly great problem solver and researcher ad-nauseum. For almost twenty years in the oil & gas industry, I analyzed data to solve problems. I compared graphs and flowcharts to understand what was happening in a system and I even helped lead root cause failure analysis when there were significant problems. In 2016, I became my most important, and difficult, problem ever to solve. And what I discovered over the next six years was shocking.

Sure, the high amounts of stress I was under for years was definitely not healthy nor was the toxic environment I worked in daily. But what about the chronic levels of inflammation I had been battling, the low level infections my body had to fight daily, the suboptimal Vitamin D? What about all of these clues my body had been giving me that were just ignored? What IF they had been addressed sooner rather than later? Maybe I wouldn't have lost so much of life along the way, so many years and decisions dictated by my failing health and handfuls of pills.

If I could tell you just three things to shift your health in a positive direction, the number one thing I would tell you is to spend 10-15 minutes of your early morning outdoors soaking up the light without sunglasses and exposing as much skin as you possibly can. Bonus points if you are barefoot in the grass. There is a ton of science behind doing this that would take me more than two pages to explain but this is so beneficial for your body. From resetting your circadian rhythm to strengthening your immune system, this is one of the best things you can implement into your daily lifestyle and it's FREE!

The second thing I would tell you is to check several bloodwork markers in the labs that you already have that often get overlooked and could be key to helping you understand why you are feeling exhausted all the time. The top markers I would have you check are calcium and/or Vitamin D. If your calcium is lower than 9.2 and/or your Vitamin D level is below 80, then you should add in a good quality Vitamin D3 supplement for optimal health. Vitamin D3 with K2 is best for absorption but be sure and check with your doctor first.

I would also have you check your sodium and potassium levels. For optimal, healthy bodies, I prefer to have sodium in the range 135-140 mmol/L and potassium in the range 4.0-4.5 mmol/L. For either of these markers, anything above or below could indicate a stressed adrenal that needs a little TLC.

The last thing I would tell you is to take a moment and observe the environment where you spend the most amount of time every day. For many of us, that is the place where we work. How is the air quality? If it's not good, consider investing in an air filter for your work space. What is the quality of your drinking water? Again, if it's not good quality water, consider investing in a water filter. Are you drinking enough water? For most people, my recommendation is one-half the body weight in water. So if you weigh 150 lbs., you should aim to hydrate your body with ~75 ounces of water. If you're wondering, that's just over 4.5 water bottles.

Small, simple changes like these are sustainable over the long haul and have the potential to create significant shifts during a lifetime. Shifts that allow you to continue working and excelling in your career, being the spouse/parent/grandparent that you dream about, and prevent you from becoming a statistic. You can find me at www. thefxnclinic.com/shift or on Facebook at The FxN Clinic.

* * *

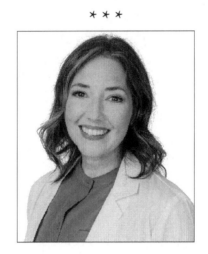

Julie Richard, FNS-BC, FMS, CNAS, CNS

CHAPTER 16:

Weight Loss Resistance: There Is An Answer!

By: Dr. Lisa D'Eramo

You are doing EVERYTHING that conventional wisdom tells you to do to lose weight plus trying all the fad diets, cleanses, and supplement regimes with no success. Scratching your head in frustration and anger, moving on to trying the next gimmick or just giving up because "You are of that age where weight loss doesn't happen." Know that the answer isn't necessarily eating less, a specific diet, or exercising more. You are doing enough. You aren't lying to yourself with all of your efforts. The real underlying cause hasn't been revealed to you yet.

Here are the five most common issues doctors, coaches, or your trainer aren't taking into consideration or looking at to correct your weight loss resistance issues.

1. Overtraining or not eating enough/right balance of food (macronutrients).

Many of us decrease our calorie intake because that is what everyone tells us to do. Yes, we can't overeat, but we need enough fuel to build our muscles and to keep our metabolism strong. Consuming too few calories can cause your resting metabolic rate to slow down, thus burning fewer calories throughout the day. Also, not consuming enough protein can lead to the breakdown of your muscles and deregulate several weight-regulating hormones.

Overtraining, on the other hand, can cause chronic inflammation and an imbalance in testosterone (yes, for us women too) and cortisol leading to muscle loss, excess belly fat, and weight gain leading to weight loss resistance.

2. Hormonal Imbalances

Hormone imbalances can come from many forms or a combination of them. The most common culprits are female/male sex hormones, Thyroid, Adrenal, Insulin and Leptin/Ghrelin imbalances.

We commonly see these hormones are either not being tested, not tested in their entirety, or not analyzed correctly.

For example, when testing for Thyroid issues, most doctors look at Thyroid Stimulating Hormone (TSH) and, if you're lucky, T4. That only gives you a tiny picture of what your Thyroid is doing. TSH isn't truly a thyroid test, it's a pituitary hormone acting on your Thyroid. You need to have at least seven to nine tests for you to get the full Thyroid picture. TSH, T3, T4, T3 Uptake, Free T3, Free T4, Reverse T3, and additionally Thyroid Peroxidase Antibodies and Thyroglobulin Antibodies.

3. Toxins

Toxins that disrupt the body's natural metabolism and hormone balance are called obesogens. These chemicals come from everyday items such as plastics, artificial scents, Teflon cookware, mold, pesticides, cosmetics, food additives and heavy metals like aluminum and mercury. All of these and more can cause background inflammation messing with hormone balance and causing weight gain and the inability to lose weight.

Environmental toxins (along with chronic stress, an unhealthy diet or food sensitivities) can also create dysbiosis or gut imbalances, which eventually develop into problems like leaky gut. Those problems put your immune system in overdrive and increase inflammation, creating a vicious cycle that feeds weight loss resistance.

4. Stress

Stress can be mental, emotional or physical. Stress triggers the release of hormones like cortisol that increase abdominal fat and slows metabolism making it harder to release weight. Cortisol is responsible for regulating how much sugar (glucose) and fat gets stored in your body, and how much is released to use for fuel. Also, stress can cause biochemical and other hormonal changes that lead to abnormal eating habits.

5. Sleep

Adults who sleep less than seven hours per night are more likely to have weight issues than people who can sleep more. When you don't get enough sleep your body releases cortisol which you remember, can increase abdominal fat and slow metabolism. When cortisol is elevated, it can also lead to an increase in your blood glucose level and insulin level which can devastate weight loss efforts. Also, a lack of sleep causes the hormone Ghrelin to increase. Ghrelin is the primary hunger hormone and causes you to feel hungry even when you don't need to eat.

Some actions that you can currently and easily incorporate into your lifestyle to correct weight loss resistance are:

1. Prioritizing protein and fiber in your diet. Eat whole foods as much as possible.

2. Lift weights instead of doing long cardio workouts. More muscle equals higher metabolism. Hours of cardio can be stressful for some individuals causing an increase in your levels of cortisol. Combine walking, yoga and/or breath work if stress is a component.

3. Work on finding and decreasing stress (physical, emotional, or mental sources) and improving sleep hygiene.

4. Look for hidden toxins in your environment and remove them. Especially plastics in the kitchen; artificial fragrances in soaps, air fresheners, candles; and preservatives in packaged foods.

Feeling stuck is overwhelming and frustrating. Dr. Lisa and the other practitioners at her office can help you with many conditions finding the underlying root cause using a combination of holistic, naturopathic, foundational, and functional medicine that is individualized for each patient. Contact us now to take a deep dive into your health and wellness to become the best, youthful, and healthiest version of yourself!

You can learn more about her and Pathways Center at www. PC4HW.com or call the office at 630.323.2400. We accept local in-person and long-distance virtual clients.

✶ ✶ ✶

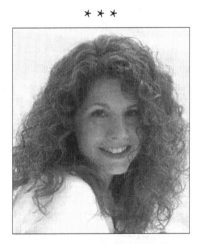

Dr. Lisa D'Eramo is the senior clinician and director of Pathways Center for Health and Wellness in Hinsdale, Illinois. She was driven to holistic health after seeing how the traditional medical system did not have the answer to her autoimmune diseases, which have been in remission for over twenty years using the natural medicine approach.

CHAPTER 17:

Heal Your Sleep Deprivation Rollercoaster

By: Dr. Christine Cantwell DC

If you're like me, you've been on the sleep deprivation rollercoaster, relying on external substances to manage sleepless nights. In midlife, I found myself questioning why I had worked so hard to build a successful career and family life, only to feel exhausted, foggy, and depressed all the time. **Does this routine sound familiar?**

- **7:00 am**: Coffee, lots of it—my reason for being at this moment.
- **11:30 am and 3:30 pm**: Sugary treats in the mid-morning and afternoon.
- **5:30-8:30 pm**: Wine to wind down with dinner, and after!
- **11:00 pm**: Benadryl or Unisom at bedtime to hopefully sleep through the night. And repeat…

I was a self-employed health professional, a late-in-life mother at forty-three, a part of the "sandwich" generation, and then how about living through a global pandemic for extra stress? For years I did not sleep well. Talking with my patients, I know you have been there too.

Even with blessings like a supportive partner, a secure home, and a flexible work schedule, I felt the weight of being the "default" parent and handling the emotional and logistical labor of the household. I deeply resonated with the meme: "If you ever wonder what Mom is doing, Mom's doing everything."

My child was a good sleeper, but while he would fall back asleep easily after waking at night to nurse, I couldn't. My alertness at 3 a.m. was through the roof, and no amount of calming meditations helped. My frustration grew when well-meaning comments like, "No one sleeps well with little kids," dismissed my struggles. It felt like a failure; my child slept fine, so why couldn't I?

Lack of quality sleep bled into other areas of my health. Who has the energy to exercise when you're exhausted? I'd start routines with temporary motivation but would get sick immediately due to depletion. My weight was steadily increasing, and so were my A1C and cholesterol levels, and not too shockingly my liver enzymes were also elevated.

Tracking my sleep with devices only added to my frustration. Biofeedback, cooling blankets, grounding sheets, and meditation apps offered no relief. I hoped for a magic bullet, but chronic use of antihistamines such as Benadryl literally shrinks your brain and increases the likelihood of dementia.

I learned that consistent sleep between 1 and 4 a.m. is essential for our brain's natural opiate receptors to replenish themselves and function properly. No wonder I had a diminished ability to experience joy, and was deepening the cycle of reliance on stimulants and sedatives to feel "okay" and get by.

Frustrated with lack of help from my MD, my problems weren't at a level they could diagnose me with a disease, yet! I took a deep dive into functional medicine. As a practitioner, I ordered my own blood work, gut tests and hormone panels and slowly put the pieces together, first for myself and then for my patients who suffered similarly.

Here are the **5 Keys of Body, Mind, and Spirit** to heal your "Sleep Axis":

1. **Chronic Infections**: Address hidden infections affecting the gut-brain axis. Parasites often become active at night, and subclinical infections (like bad bacteria and candida) can cause sugar and alcohol cravings. Chronic constipation and poor gut motility can lead to toxin buildup, overwhelming your detox system.

2. **Neurochemical Balance**: Test your Cortisol Awakening Response and get a complete thyroid panel. Targeted nutritional supplements can make a big difference. Adaptogens may help, but need to be chosen based on your specific biochemistry. A comprehensive 3-4 month protocol is key to healing cellular and glandular depletion. It takes at least one month per year you have been experiencing the symptoms as a guideline. So in my case, six months.

3. **Trauma Release**: Treat sleep issues like a phobia. Fear of waking at night can create anxiety and perpetuate the cycle. Tension & Trauma Release Exercises (TRE) are effective in releasing stress without years of talk therapy. You can do these exercises with a facilitator or online tutorials.

4. **Structural Changes**: Focus on changing your wake-up routine, not your bedtime. Wake up early (around 5 a.m.) for ten days to reset your natural sleep rhythm. This will initially be challenging but will help you catch the first wave of sleep onset at night. Invest in earplugs, a king-sized bed, and separate blankets to minimize disturbances from loved ones.

5. **Kick the Sugar and Alcohol to the curb**: Start moving for thirty minutes a day, and get ready to eliminate or reduce alcohol and refined sugars. Address the underlying stressors first; it's not a lack of willpower but digestive dysfunction, chronic infections and hormonal imbalances

that make cravings feel irresistible. With better nutrient reserves, balanced cortisol, and reduced body tension, making healthier choices becomes easier and more sustainable.

These days I do sleep like a baby, at least 90% of the time, and when I don't, I know it won't be an ongoing plague and I have the tools to get back on track in short order. Sleep quality is truly foundational to healing and it is often the first step in tackling many other health challenges. Take the time to heal this issue and it will pay you back many times over, plus you can actually enjoy the life you have worked so hard for all these years.

* * *

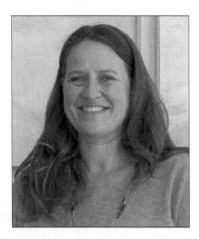

Dr. Christine Cantwell DC has cared for thousands of families, over the last twenty years as a chiropractor in private practice. Known for her compassion and depth of knowledge, she holds certifications in Trauma Releasing Exercises (TRE), is a Functional Blood Work specialist, from the Aperion Epigenetic Academy and is FMA certified in Functional Medicine.

As a mother later in life, Dr. Cantwell has faced health challenges like insomnia, exhaustion, metabolic and neuroendocrine imbalances. Seeking solutions for herself and others, she expanded her practice to include personalized functional medicine, offering tailored solutions to address underlying imbalances and bridging the gap where conventional approaches fall short.

She can be reached at: www.drchristinecantwell.com

CHAPTER 18:

Harnessing Generations Of Healing: A Journey To Wholeness

By: Bonnie Ridge, FNP-BC, CTP, BC-FMP, BC-FHC

Imagine waking up every morning feeling refreshed, energized and free from the chronic ailments that once tethered you to a carousel of medications. This is not a distant dream, but a reachable reality. My journey into the world of holistic health is not just a profession; it's a legacy and a personal crusade, inspired by a lineage of medical providers and fueled by my experiences as a mother and a healer.

Born into a family where medicine was the vernacular, I grew up shadowed by the towering figures of my father, a devoted physician of fifty-seven years, and my mother, a skilled surgical nurse and midwife. Their dedication to health was profound, yet traditional. My path, however, diverged into a realization that would reshape my understanding of healing. With over a decade of experience in hospitals and primary care as a nurse and nurse practitioner, I came face-to-face with a disheartening truth: conventional medicine's reliance on pharmaceuticals often fell short of truly healing my patients.

The real turning point came from a deeply personal challenge. As a mother of two children with life-threatening food allergies, the battle to safeguard their health opened my eyes to the pivotal role of diet and environment in our wellbeing. The quest to eliminate processed foods and identify toxic daily exposures was more than enlightening—it was transformative. This hands-on battle against hidden dangers revealed to me the critical missing pieces in modern healthcare.

Today, armed with this knowledge, I guide my patients on a transformative journey towards true health. We begin with comprehensive advanced testing to identify obstacles to healing, followed by dietary adjustments that replace harmful substances with nourishing, organic whole foods. But our approach does not stop at nutrition. We incorporate mindfulness, physical activity, and supplement support to create a balanced, thriving existence.

Your Steps Toward a Healthier Tomorrow

You, too, can embark on this path to rejuvenation and vitality. Start by making simple yet impactful changes in your daily life. Introduce more whole foods into your diet, focusing on organic produce to reduce exposure to harmful pesticides and chemicals. Evaluate your environment: replace plastic containers with glass to avoid chemical leachates and eliminate synthetic fragrances that pervade many homes and personal care products.

Moreover, embracing activities that reduce stress and improve physical health is crucial. Commit to regular physical exercise, which not only strengthens the body but also clears the mind. Ensure adequate sleep—at least eight hours per night—to allow your body to repair, restore, and rejuvenate. These practices are not just adjustments; they are investments in a healthier, more vibrant you.

As we stand on the shoulders of medical giants, let us not be confined by the limits of past practices. Instead, let us expand the definition of healing to encompass all aspects of our lives, making informed, mindful choices that honor our bodies and our environment. Join me in this holistic health revolution, where every small change contributes to a monumental improvement in our quality of life. Together, we can transform not just our health, but our future.

My mission is to help individuals who are ready to partner with me for guidance on their journey to healing themselves. I want to empower you to optimize your whole body, mind, and spirit so you can feel your best from the inside out and thrive! Book a call with me today! You can find me at Integrative & Functional Health (www. integrativeandfunctionalhealth.com) or at Renew Integrative Wellness (www.renewintegrativewellness.com).

* * *

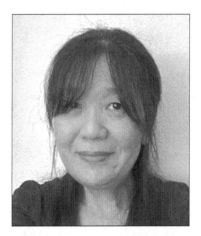

Bonnie Ridge, FNP-BC, CTP, BC-FMP, BC-FHC and Foundational Medicine Specialist

Bonnie Ridge is a Board-Certified Family Nurse Practitioner, Certified Trauma Professional, Board-Certified Functional Medicine Practitioner, and Board-Certified Functional Health Coach. Most recently, she has been certified as a Foundational Medicine Specialist. She has completed all courses at The Institute for Functional Medicine, Functional Medicine for Nurses, Functional Nurse Academy, Functional Diagnostic Nutrition, Functional Medicine Academy, and The Institute for Integrative Nutrition. As a 4th generation medical professional with over a decade of experience in the healthcare field, she values every chance to assist those in need and to positively impact the lives of others. She is the founder of Integrative & Functional Health and co-founder of Renew Integrative Wellness, both virtual practices in California. She specializes in gut and brain health, food allergy and sensitivity, and the analysis of blood chemistry lab results to optimize health. She also has a passion for finding solutions in relational trauma and addiction for overall well-being.

CHAPTER 19:

From Zero to Hero: A short story about the physically ill, suicidal person, who completely healed himself and became blissful

By: Anthony E Scrima, Jr, DC, MSACN

The little guy had issues with his bowels. Since he was a wee, young lad he had a personal relationship with the four walls of his parent's bathroom. Always bloated after meals with gas and noise, he tried frantically to remain hidden from other people. They thought he was a loner, a loser, a freak. Isolated from the rest of the world, he was unapproachable.

He was totally embarrassed to go out in public. As time went on, he would miss days at school or at work. People noticed. His grades slipped. He crawled further into his head. Eventually, he learned how to live with it and life went on. His bosses were always upset with him and he was miserable having to go to work with this condition. So, he bounced from job to job and relationship to relationship.

The guy was seemingly distracted. He just couldn't really hold a conversation long and didn't make a lot of eye contact. Sure, he had friends, but he didn't know how to be a friend. His mind was always preoccupied with something. Was he autistic? No. He had no diagnosis. His blood labs were always good and he was always told of how healthy he was. He was just dealing with some hidden thing. No one knew.

He suffered daily with stomach pains that would have him bent over and he didn't understand why he had to deal with this any longer. There was no rhyme or reason to it. Some days he would feel completely great. Most days he would feel sleepy after eating. His family would get angry with him and they thought he was being rude. He'd disappear into a bathroom for hours when they would go out somewhere. Then he would be in and out of the bathroom on other days.

He was irritable, cranky and grumpy most of the time. No one wanted to be around him much. Then the worst part was the depression and then came the suicidal thoughts. He was angry and would lash out at the wrong people. He gained forty plus pounds of puffy disgustingness and he felt sluggish all of the time. His heartburn was relentless. Oftentimes it kept him up over the course of the night. He did this for forty plus years.

The little guy is I. Now Dr. Tony.

Finally, I couldn't take it anymore as things got progressively worse. I studied EVERYTHING nutritional, medical and experimental. It took years of my time and hundreds of thousands of dollars in research and education. The answer was stupid simple and got me to where I am today. I lost thirty-five pounds, put on some muscle mass, got stronger, healthier and continue to surprise myself. I felt so energetic. I could feel my lungs and I could breathe easier. I was excited to jump out of bed in the morning!

It's as if it were yesterday. I can completely remember that day, the day when EVERYTHING changed…

You see, one major thing I didn't know was that the intestines have their own brain and immune system! They can operate independently of the upstairs brain. You basically sit on your second brain. So, whatever is going on in either brain can effect the other one in kind. This explains the depression, the anger, the suicidal thoughts, the irritability...all of the emotions that come with it.

First, I figured out that digestion is the first system of attack when handling a not so healthy body. However, digestion doesn't start in the mouth. It actually starts in the brain! When you think about it, most humans share a custom where they pray before meals. It is typically giving thanks or being grateful for having the food they are about to eat. What this does is prepare the brain to signal the organs that it is time to release digestive chemicals to breakdown the food into its proper constituents. So, before meals I PRAY and show gratitude!

Second, I learned that rushing through meals and eating while under stress was detrimental to digestion. The food cannot breakdown properly. Blood and oxygen are shunted to where they are needed most under duress; away from the gut! Gut walls break down and allow big proteins to get in, which causes more problems. Some cultures, after prayer, will chew their food hundreds of times! This allows the surface area of the food to increase so as to be affected by the enzymes in the mouth before they continue on downstream. I now slow down and CHEW my food!

Third, I realized I had to tailor what goes into my tummy. I discovered food sensitivities. They are different from actual food allergies. It could take days for this reaction to happen, whereas, a food allergy you'd know pretty quickly. As I said, the gut has an entire immune system within it that will attack foreign particles. If your body reacts to specific foods and you are repeatedly eating the wrong foods then your immune system will go haywire. This can compromise your organs which can become dysfunctional, brain chemicals can fluctuate too greatly and a host of "unrelated" symptoms can manifest and negatively affect your life. Remember my story?

You can start praying and feeling grateful before your meals. You can start working on being calm while you eat and chew your food. You can get food sensitivity tested. We have a great FREE mini-course on food sensitivity that can help you complete your knowledge about getting tested. We have two big GIFTS for people who watch our FREE course on the website. Find out more at tummytailors.com

For me, it's all about empowering you to maximize your digestion and making you healthy again. It's only a decision away. Be thankful for this wonderful opportunity. I'm Dr. Tony with Tummy Tailors. Thank you for allowing me to share my story.

* * *

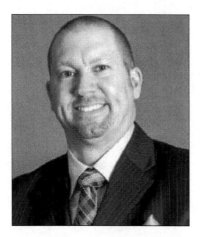

Anthony E Scrima, Jr, DC, MSACN received his Bachelor of Science degree in Exercise Science and Human Performance at UMass-Boston in 2000, his Doctor of Chiropractic degree from New York Chiropractic College in 2006 and a Master of Science in 2020 from NYCC's School of Health Sciences & Education with honors. While attending UMass-Boston, Dr. Scrima was a member of the Strategic Planning Committee in the College of Nursing, which oversaw changes in the college's infrastructure and provided access facilitation for both students and faculty. At NYCC, he interned at the University of Buffalo Medical Center, the Salvation Army and was a member of the medical team for the Men's & Women's Division 1 Track and Field Championships in New York City. Dr. Scrima is also the author of My Chiropractic Physician: For My Neck Pain, Back Pain & Beyond.

CHAPTER 20:

Fueling Your Greatness from the Inside Out: A Letter to My Teenage Athletes

By: Nicole Tatro

Dear Owen, Aidan and Ella,

As I sit down to write this letter, I can't help but think back to my own time as a competitive athlete. I played softball and field hockey at Sacred Heart University, driven by the same passion and dedication I see in each of you today. But there's something I wish I had known back then—something that could have taken me even further and saved me from the exhaustion and injuries that came from pushing my body beyond its limits. That something is understanding the power of your internal health—your internal stats—and how they hold the key to not just surviving your sport but truly thriving.

You've been raised in a family where performance, health, and recovery are everyday conversations, so it's no surprise you've already begun to understand the importance of nutrition, training, and rest. But what I want to share with you goes even deeper. It's about optimizing your body from the inside out, tuning in to what your body is telling you through things like bloodwork, DNA analysis, nutrient deficiencies, and inflammation markers—long before symptoms appear.

When I was your age, I didn't have the tools I now have at my fingertips. I didn't know that what was happening on the inside was just as important—if not more so—than what was happening on the field. My coaches pushed me to run harder, lift heavier, and play through pain, but no one ever talked about what was really going on beneath the surface.

The truth is, understanding your internal health is your competitive advantage. By staying on top of your internal stats—whether it's making sure your immune system is strong, your recovery is on point, or your muscles are being nourished at the cellular level—you can push yourself to new levels without breaking down. With the addition of DNA analysis, we now have the ability to look even deeper at how your body is uniquely wired—your genetic blueprint—and how to best support it. You'll have more energy, faster recovery times, and less injury risk, and you'll be able to stay on top of your game not just for a season but for your entire career. Your body is your most powerful asset, and taking care of it from the inside out will allow you to keep doing what you love for years to come.

You already know how much time and effort we've put into understanding how your body functions—looking at bloodwork, DNA data, customizing supplements, and fine-tuning your nutrition to support your performance goals. These are things I wish I had back when I was your age. I can only imagine how different my journey might have been had I understood the importance of nutrient timing, functional ranges, DNA insights and true recovery. And while I can't go back and rewrite my story, I'm grateful to be able to help guide yours with everything I've learned.

Quick Tips For Any Athlete:

1. **Start with Bloodwork:** If you haven't done it yet, get your bloodwork checked to know your internal stats. It's the best way to uncover deficiencies or issues before they become problems.

2. **Hydrate for Performance:** Drinking plenty of water isn't just for games or practices—consistent hydration helps your body recover and perform optimally every day.

3. **Optimize Recovery:** After intense training, prioritize sleep, protein intake, and active recovery (like stretching or foam rolling) to help your muscles repair faster.

4. **Time Your Nutrition:** Fuel your body with the right nutrients before and after workouts. Carbohydrates before activity can help with performance, while proteins and healthy fats after training help with muscle repair.

5. **Listen to Your Body:** Pay attention to the subtle signs—if something feels off, take the time to rest or adjust your training.

So, when you're feeling frustrated with the grind, when it seems like the gains are slower than you want them to be, or when everyone around you is talking about pushing harder without listening to their bodies—remember this: you have the tools. You have the knowledge. And you have the power to tap into your body's natural ability to heal, grow, and recover. Don't ever underestimate the importance of your internal stats. They are the foundation upon which everything else is built.

I'm so incredibly proud of each of you. Not just for the athletes you are, but for the amazing young people you've become. Keep listening to your bodies, keep taking care of yourselves from the inside out, and remember, your future is limitless.

With all my love and belief in your greatness,

Mom (Dr. Nicole Tatro)

P.S. For any of you reading this who want to learn more about how to optimize your performance through bloodwork, DNA analysis, natural supplementation and targeted nutrition, you can find more information at www.the-eliteathlete.com.

* * *

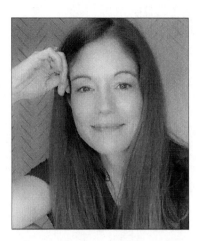

I'm **Dr. Nicole Tatro, DPT, INHC, DipACLM, PBP, PN 1+2, PHC**

I help high-level athletes unleash their peak performance by leveraging personalized bloodwork analysis and customized plans, so they can dominate their sport with fierce confidence and unstoppable energy. As a wife and mother of five, with three high-level athletes among them, I understand the dedication it takes to excel in sports. My own journey began as a competitive three-sport high school athlete and I continued to pursue my passion in college playing softball and field hockey at Sacred Heart University. Although now I am not on any organized team, I still call myself an athlete! I also coach both softball and field hockey teams in my hometown. I LOVE athletes! My personal experiences combined with my professional expertise have equipped me with a unique perspective on optimizing athletic performance. I am committed to helping athletes reach their full potential. I wish someone would have taught me what I know now when I was young and pushing towards my athletic dreams. I am doing that with my own children and want them to be the best that they possibly can while they strive towards their athletic dreams.

https://www.elitehealthandwellnessvt.com/elevateyourgame

CHAPTER 21:

How to Boost Testosterone Naturally!

By: Dr. John Olsen

Are you sick of feeling tired all the time? Do you feel like you're barely able to get through the day and then crash on the couch when you get home? Are you having a hard time focusing? Maybe thinking good luck asking me what I did three weekends ago because I don't remember. These could all be symptoms of low testosterone and an underlying issue that needs help. Imagine waking up each morning with boundless energy, a sharp mind, and the physical strength to tackle any challenge! Natural testosterone boosting is the key to transforming your health and living life to the fullest. Hi, I am Dr. John Olsen, a chiropractic physician, foundational blood work specialist and overall advocate for natural healing therapies.

My journey towards discovering the power of natural testosterone boosting began with a personal health crisis. As I reached the age of forty, I found myself starting to struggle with many of the issues I listed above. Many of my peers in the medical field told me that my testosterone was probably low and that I should get testosterone replacement therapy!

As these symptoms started to show more in me, I began to feel like a tired old grandpa trying to climb Mt. Everest! I felt like I was hitting a brick wall every morning just trying to get out of bed. My drive in life and business began to decline, and it took everything I had just to grind out the day. My ability to problem-solve became terrible, I wanted to avoid all stressful situations. So, even though I had lived my life without being on any prescriptions, I started to consider getting testosterone therapy. So then I started to research the side effects of going on TRT and thought, there has to be another way! No, I don't want a greater risk for blood clots, possible prostate issues and shrinking testicles just to name a few of them.

I set out on a journey to educate myself with some of the leading functional blood work specialists in the country, quickly realizing that healthy people have a more narrow, "optimal" range in their blood work. This became my passion: to interpret blood work for patients through a different lens. What I found through this journey is that there is definitely another path. This path doesn't make pharmaceutical companies millions of dollars, but it requires the accountability of a man who wants to take control of his health, to facilitate a better-functioning hormonal pathway and avoid all the risk factors that come with TRT. This is how I became known as Dr T Booster! I developed a ninety-day natural testosterone boosting program which includes one of the most important things you can do on this journey, get extensive blood work and have it analyzed by a practitioner that understands functional medicine.

I can't tell you how much my life has changed by incorporating the protocols I have put together in this program. I started waking up in the morning feeling rested, calm and in a much more positive mood. I felt ready to tackle the tasks of the day. Physically my body fat began to decrease! My gym lifting sessions started to produce an increase in my muscle mass size. Overall my body is functioning at a more optimal level without having the side effects of TRT!

These experiences, both personal and professional, fueled my passion for helping others achieve optimal health through natural methods. Research shows that men's testosterone levels have been declining steadily over the past few decades due to lifestyle and environmental factors. In fact, over the past twenty years the average testosterone has dropped nearly thirty percent! This decline contributes to a range of health issues, from fatigue and depression to decreased muscle mass and increased body fat. Natural testosterone boosting isn't just about overcoming symptoms; it's about reclaiming your life!

So, what can you do now to start boosting your testosterone naturally you might ask? Here are three science-backed tips straight from my Dr T Booster Program to help you begin your journey:

1. Optimize Your Diet

Incorporate Nutrient-Rich Foods: Focus on foods high in zinc and Vitamin D, such as lean meats, fish, nuts and leafy green vegetables. These nutrients are essential for testosterone production. Diet is critical and I go into more detail with food and its effects on testosterone in my program.

Healthy Fats: Incorporate sources of healthy fats like avocados, nuts, seeds and olive oil, which are essential for hormone synthesis.

2. Exercise Regularly

Engage in Resistance Training: Lifting weights and other forms of resistance training 2-3 times per week are proven to stimulate testosterone production.

High-Intensity Interval Training (HIIT): Short bursts of intense activity followed by recovery periods can boost testosterone levels more effectively than steady-state cardio.

3. Prioritize Sleep

You need 7-9 Hours of Quality Sleep: Sleep is crucial for hormone production. Ensure you get enough rest each night to support your body's natural testosterone production. Excessive exposure to blue light from screens before bedtime can disrupt sleep and circadian rhythms, indirectly affecting testosterone levels.

Maintain a Consistent Sleep Schedule: Going to bed and waking up at the same time each day can improve sleep quality and overall health.

By incorporating these strategies into your daily routine, you can start seeing improvements in your energy, mood and overall health. Remember, natural testosterone boosting is a journey, and consistency is key. Take the first step today and embrace a healthier, more vibrant you!

✳ ✳ ✳

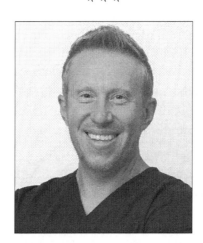

You can find this program at www.drtbooster.com; to a more fulfilling life, **Dr. John Olsen.**

CHAPTER 22:

Which Came First: The Chicken or the Egg?

By: Hali Laricey, CFNC, CFBS

I remember having this discussion with my grandparents as a very young child. It's an age-old question that has been debated by children and adults alike. This well-known metaphor is used to describe a situation when cause and effect are unclear.

I like to ask my clients a similar question when we start working together. Which came first, your symptom or your condition?

Most of the time, I get a deer-in-the-headlights look, or a stutter, or an, "I don't know." My goal is to stimulate some thought about the current condition we are discussing. It's important to consider this.

To be honest and transparent here, my question is rhetorical in nature. What I want to accomplish is a shift in the mindset when it comes to thinking about taking our health back. Are we seeking a diagnosis so we can, then, treat the illness? Do we believe that a diagnosis, or a label, will finally name the problem that the doctors can fix?

Let's back things up for a minute and ask this question instead. Where exactly does disease begin?

More than 2000 years ago, Hippocrates suggested that all disease begins in the gut. I believe he was correct, and this premise is the foundation of my practice. Increasing evidence shows that many chronic, systemic, metabolic diseases do, in fact, begin in the gut. The gut bacteria and the integrity of the gut lining strongly affect your health. Sound complicated? It's not! And you don't need expensive functional medicine tests to find out if your gut needs help. I can tell by looking at your Comprehensive Metabolic Panel (CMP) that your doctor runs annually. These results are probably sitting in your portal right now and can tell us immediate details about numerous things going on in your body. In fact, the normal labs your doctor orders like the CBC, lipids, A1C, iron, hormone, and thyroid panels hold a wealth of knowledge about you and your health that is waiting to be uncovered.

If we can back everything up and get the gut healthy, then everything else in your body has a chance to reset to a state of homeostasis. I want to help people realize this BEFORE they get a diagnosis, before things get off the charts, before certain genes get turned on, and before symptoms become debilitating. I'm a believer. I believe this is possible. I've seen it with my own eyes! And seeing people take their lives and their health back is the best feeling in the world!

I have seen my approach work for people suffering from mystery symptoms and autoimmune conditions. I have also achieved great success with the aging population who just want to grow older gracefully and avoid doctors, specialists, medications, expensive treatments, and tests if possible. My approach works for the chronically sick as well as anyone looking for optimal health, whatever their stage in life.

If you are currently suffering from a mystery illness or an autoimmune condition, you are not alone. Both groups make up the largest category of chronic illnesses. More than 80% of those suffering is female. Shockingly, most of these patients see at least four doctors over 3-7 years before getting a diagnosis. What is happening to their bodies during that 3-7 years while they wait for an answer? In addition, these conditions can place a considerable burden on healthcare budgets.

What if you had someone in your toolkit you could call to review your labs and any symptoms you're dealing with and put together a plan to support the systems in your body that might be suffering some deficiencies? I'm virtually raising my hand right now and inviting you to add me to your toolkit!

Our healthcare system has not kept pace with the health of the patients it was created to serve. I love doctors. I believe in medical intervention, especially for acute care. If I'm in a car accident and bleeding, then I want the best triage doctors in the country working on me. But when it comes to chronic care, two-thirds of doctors feel inadequately trained in the care of the chronically ill. Specialists are generally unaware of autoimmune diseases or advances in treatment outside their area of specialty.

The work I do provides answers to suffering people. Today, I help people feel better by looking at the complete picture of their health and well-being. I view everyone as a whole person, made up of cells, organs, tissues, glands, and systems that all work together. Each entity was wonderfully made to be healthy, strong, and age gracefully. Diagnoses and symptoms are labels, not identities or destinations.

I will leave you with this tip. To find out if you have a leaky digestive system, grab your Comprehensive Metabolic Panel lab results. Look for these three markers and ranges. If your lab values fall outside these ranges, consider slowly adding some fermented foods to your diet. Then consider talking with me. I can help: Total Protein: 6.9-7.4, Albumin: 4.0-5.0, Globulin: 2.4 - 2.8. If any marker falls outside the range, I invite you to schedule a Free Wellness Empowerment Session with me now! I hope to see you soon! (https://www.halilaricey.com/schedule)

* * *

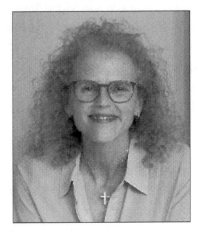

Hali Laricey, CFNC, CFBS

Functional Wellness and Nutrition Specialist

Functional Wellness with Hali

Website: halilaricey.com

Facebook: facebook.com/functionalwellnesswithhali

Instagram: instagram.com/functionalwellnesswithhali/

Call/Text: 770-530-587

Made in the USA
Columbia, SC
13 February 2025

53718630R00065